To Tim

Ready for a ... you ...

Happy Christmas

with love from
Sue xxx

Dec 2005

CW00894159

THE WORLD'S FITTEST YOU

THE WORLD'S FITTEST YOU

Four Weeks to Total Fitness

JOE DECKER

with Eric Neuhaus

DUTTON

Published by Penguin Group (USA) Inc.
375 Hudson Street, New York, New York 10014, U.S.A.
Penguin Books Ltd, Registered Offices: 80 Strand, London WC2R 0RL, England
Penguin Books Australia Ltd, 250 Camberwell Road, Camberwell,Victoria 3124, Australia
Penguin Books Canada Ltd, 10 Alcorn Avenue, Toronto, Ontario, Canada M4V 3B2
Penguin Books (N.Z.) Ltd, Cnr Rosedale and Airborne Roads,
Albany, Auckland 1310, New Zealand

Published by Dutton, a member of Penguin Group (USA) Inc.

First printing, January 2004
10   9   8   7   6   5   4   3   2   1

LIBRARY OF CONGRESS CATALOGING-IN-PUBLICATION DATA HAS BEEN APPLIED FOR.

ISBN: 0-525-94759-0

Printed in the United States of America
Set in Sabon, with accents in Trade Gothic and display in Corporate
Designed by BTDNYC

CONTENTS

INTRODUCTION

FROM FAT TO FITTEST:
BECOMING THE WORLD'S FITTEST MAN

I looked over at the bright red lights glaring from the digital clock next to my bed: 6:00 A.M. I had hardly gotten any sleep last night. Truthfully, I had just fallen asleep after three days of nonstop partying. I dragged myself out of bed and stared at myself in the mirror. I couldn't believe what I looked like. And I felt like hell. My eyes were puffed up, swollen and red, almost popping out of my sunken, ashen, white face. The rest of my body was in no better shape. My head was throbbing from the huge meal and cocktails I had whipped up the night before. I was a wreck. I really couldn't believe that reflection was me. How had I gotten here and how was I going to escape?

Looking in the mirror I disliked the image I saw. On top of that I felt aimless and without purpose in life. I was living in a dingy room in the heart of New Orleans with no career or direction to keep me going. I was depressed and felt my life had amounted to nothing. I had hit rock bottom. I did the only thing I could think of doing. I picked up the phone and called my parents for help.

That's one thing about my parents. They were always there for me. From my lowest point, there, in New Orleans, on the verge of self-destruction, to my highest achievement, which I'll tell you about later, becoming the World's Fittest Man, I never lost touch with my family and my farm-town roots. You'll see—I may be the World's Fittest Man now, but I started out as nothing more than a chubby farm boy.

I grew up in central Illinois, in a small town called Cuba. Cuba has a population of about fourteen hundred, if you count the cats and dogs too. Most people either farmed or worked at a factory. It was a great place to grow up but definitely not a very fitness- or health-conscious area. Life in Cuba was simple—just one bar, one gas station, and a general store.

My parents, Daniel and Diane, and my three younger brothers all were raised in an old farmhouse. It was very primitive living. In the winter things got so bad that the pipes would sometimes freeze and my brothers and I would play with Weeble Wobbles on the frozen bathtub or toilet. It was during these cold winter months that we would have to use an outhouse. A wood-burning stove was our only source of heat, so all of us would sleep in the same room for warmth. We would hang blankets over the doorways and throw the mattresses on the floor. I actually liked the closeness of it all.

We all worked hard around the house and on the farm to survive. All of it wasn't so bad, except when the temperature dipped to twenty below. Then, milking the cows and chopping the wood at five in the morning wasn't so much fun. It was a downright pain in the ass. My dad worked hard at the local Caterpillar factory and farmed most of his life, and my mom was a custodian at the local grade school. They are the hardest-working people I have ever met and I think that's where I got most of my drive and determination.

We always enjoyed big family suppers and breakfasts together, the kind you'd probably see on *The Waltons*. Unfortunately, most of those big meals were filled with fat and lard. My mom was a great cook, but she didn't think too much about fat content or calories. Our typical meals were nice big juicy steaks, fried chicken, and my favorite, biscuits and gravy. Lots of bacon grease, which was kept on the stove in a can, and Crisco fried foods. As you can imagine, all that kind of food made me a chubby boy.

It never seemed fair to me that I was the chubby one and my brothers were thin and lean. They seemed never to gain weight. Why were they so thin and I so chubby? That question drove me crazy, but it made me more determined to work harder at getting myself in shape.

The school bus was the worst. Since my brothers were younger, they could do little to stop the older kids who teased and taunted me about my weight. I vowed somehow to lose the weight one day and get even with those older guys on the bus.

Things changed when I got to high school. I used my "extra" weight to excel at powerlifting and then slimmed down to play football and run track. As I became more popular, I also made honor roll just about every semester. Losing those extra pounds really boosted my self-confidence. No longer was I the chubby boy who got picked on but an athlete who excelled on the football field and in the classroom. But all of that changed in an instant.

In my senior year I suffered a really bad football injury. My left calf got smashed up after a few hard smacks. All the nerves were so damaged that I couldn't feel anything from the knee down. At first the doctors thought it was just a bruise but then realized the damage was much more severe—so severe that they considered amputation. Luckily for me they figured out it was anterior compartment syndrome. They sliced a thirteen-inch incision down my calf to release the pressure and finally ordered me on crutches for a couple of months.

The unlucky part is that those few months kept me off the football field and in front of the television. Not surprisingly, that was a formula for rapid weight gain. I packed on over thirty pounds, consuming mostly pizza, Twinkies, and Coca-Cola. In so little time I had become the unhappy "fat boy" again. More than anything, I was depressed. The football scholarship that I had hoped would be my ticket to college and out of small-town Cuba suddenly disappeared. It was like my worst nightmare had come true and I couldn't wake myself up to stop it.

Since my parents couldn't afford college without the help of a scholarship, I decided to join the army right after graduating from high school. I planned to pay for college after a short stint in the military. I was shipped off to Fort Benning, Georgia, eager to start my basic training. What I hadn't planned for next was failing my first army physical-fitness test. Those months on the sofa eating nothing but junk food had left me in awful physical shape. I could barely do ten push-ups and I huffed and puffed through a two-mile run. I was just about crawling the last stretch. I felt like Bill Murray's character in that hilarious movie *Stripes*. But what was happening to me wasn't a comedy at all. It was the worst kind of tragedy. My drill sergeant ordered me into the unofficial military "fat-boy program."

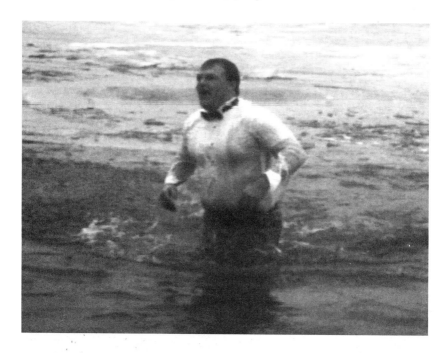

As you can imagine, being eighteen and sent off with all the other military physical-fitness failures was completely humiliating and embarrassing. I was even too ashamed to write home to my parents. I was their first boy to move out of the house on my own, so they had high expectations for me. More than anything I didn't want to let them down. What a disappointment it would have been for them to learn of my failure.

So while all the other recruits were relaxing after dinner or on weekends, I was out there working my butt off doing extra push-ups, sit-ups, pull-ups. And that's no joke. For meals all the "fat boys" were placed on a special eating program different from the rest of the recruits'. Cottage cheese, fruit, and salad were some of our staples. I remember looking over at the desserts the others were enjoying. Once I got so tempted I couldn't stop myself. One of the drill sergeants learned of my unhealthy indiscretion and punished me with more push-ups (above and beyond the extra we did anyway).

Let me tell you this, that weight didn't just melt away. I'm sorry to tell you that no magic pill or crazy diet got me back in shape. What did was lots of hard work, sweat, and commitment. I set a goal and really stuck to it. I worked hard to lose every single pound. Nothing came easy. But eventually I did it. I passed the next physical fitness test with flying colors and proudly joined the other recruits.

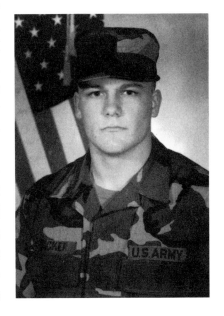

After my three years of service with the 10th Mountain Division in Fort Drum, New York, I headed off to pursue my real dream, college. I moved back to Illinois and enrolled in a prelaw program at Western Illinois University.

After two years at college I became disillusioned and restless. I guess it's pretty common to feel that way. I didn't want to be a lawyer and wasn't quite sure what I wanted to do with my life. I figured some time off might help me decide.

I packed up my bags, tossed them in the back of my white Ford pickup truck, and roamed around the country. Eventually, I ended up in New Orleans working as a bartender. If you're a tourist, New Orleans is a great place to visit because the party on Bourbon Street never stops. It's Mardi Gras twenty-four hours a day, 365 days a year. If you happen to live and work on Bourbon Street, it's easy to find yourself in the center of that never-ending party. And that's exactly what happened to me.

If you haven't figured it out by now, I'm pretty much an all-or-nothing kind of guy. Without a real focus like the army or school, I turned to eating and partying excessively. So when it came to partying, I became the best partier in New Orleans. I partied hard—so hard my friends had a nickname for me. They called me the "Mess" because I had no self-control or discipline. Working as a bartender at some of the wildest bars like the Bourbon Pub and Razoos didn't help either. I'd get off work, have a few drinks, then start partying, sometimes for three days straight when I had a few days off. During these partying binges I hardly ate. I'd sleep for a day or so and then eat nothing but pizza, hamburgers, and french fries. The whole thing became a horrible, vicious cycle. I'd feel great when I was "flying" on partying and food, but then I'd come down and crash really hard, like falling out of a ten-story window. The only way I could get myself up and off the ground again was to perpetuate the cycle.

My lifestyle was killing my body from the inside out. I had no hope or integrity. The only thing keeping me going was my family. They left many messages on my answering machine, begging me to come home. "Joe, we love you and care about you. Please come home." Those words still echo in my mind. I could have been just another statistic. "Partied till Death." I imagined it might say something like that on my tombstone. The next day I packed my things and drove back to Illinois.

When I got back home, I had very serious lifestyle choices to confront. Emotionally, I had become dependent on overeating, bingeing on alcohol, and other destructive behavior to fill some of the voids in my life. After being dependent for so many years on a self-destructive way of life, I didn't know what to do. I needed something to replace the hole in my life once filled by excessive behavior. That's when I discovered fitness.

I guess you could say what happened next led me on a path that I believe saved my life. In New Orleans I had fallen into some really awful eating habits. A typical dinner for me was thirty or forty chicken wings at Hooters, washed down with a few pitchers of beer. Other days I ate those "blooming fried onions" at Outback and nachos and potato skins loaded with just about every fattening topping. I knew that had to change if I wanted to feel and look better. I bought a low-fat-cooking book from Wal-Mart and before I knew it I was cooking my own meals with lean meats and lots of fruits and vegetables. I also filled my body with lots of water. Up until that point the only water I drank was melted ice from soda or alcohol.

At the same time I started to work out slowly at home with just an old weight set from Wal-Mart, a chin-up bar, and an old pair of beat-up running shoes. Nothing fancy, just the basics to get me going. I also started a program of walking, just a few blocks at first, then gradually building my way up to a jog, then a run. After a few months I finished my first 5K race. What a great feeling that was. The feeling I was getting from working out was keeping me sane and functioning in society. Not only that, I was building self-confidence and a sense of achievement in my life. Without fitness, I can honestly say, I'd be on a road to nowhere.

Because fitness had changed my life, I knew there were others out there I could help too. I earned my bachelor's degree in exercise science with an emphasis in corporate wellness at Western Illinois University. From there, I moved to Washington, D.C., and started my own personal training company called Body Construction, with the help of two close friends, Greg and Karen Jenkins. It was a wonderful experience, sharing in other people's fitness achievements. Later in the book you'll meet some of the people whose lives I helped turn around.

As I told you before, that addictive personality of mine—the one that got me into trouble in New Orleans—loves to take things to the extreme. Now that I had found a way to channel my energy into fitness, I needed something to stay on track. For me it's not enough just to go to the gym and work out, although that works just fine for many people. I needed a fitness challenge to keep pushing myself. Not only that, but I wanted to separate myself from the pack. I wanted to actually practice what I preached to my clients. There's nothing more satisfying than setting a new goal—whether it's finishing a race or shedding a few pounds—and then achieving it.

I started with marathons. From there I went on to try a 50-mile run. The first one, the JFK 50 Miler, was a killer. I was ill prepared and undertrained—boy, did I pay for it afterward. I was almost bedridden for the next month. If you think that 50 miles sounds crazy, just wait until you hear what I tried next. It's called the Badwater 135 and there's a reason they call it "bad." The race is 135 miles and runs through the hottest part of the United States: Death Valley, California. There, temperatures can reach up to a blistering 130 degrees during the day.

That intense heat really took its toll on my body. By the end of the first day of this grueling, nearly two-day race, I was completely dehydrated. Even though I was drinking water like a fish—about five gallons' worth sloshing around in my gut—what I hadn't considered was salt. Because I was sweating so much from the heat, I was losing all the salt in my body and my electrolytes were totally out of whack. My head felt like it was going to explode. My feet were throbbing. I was hallucinating, staggering, and stumbling—taking as many steps to the side as I was forward. A fellow runner passed me and said I was in dire need of salt. But where was I going to get salt in the middle of the desert? Luckily, my quick-thinking crew—my brother Shag and my friend Yukon—found a bottle of Morton's salt in a nearby town. When they returned I started eating the salt right out of the box. Who would have thought an ordinary box of Morton's salt could have saved my life?

At mile forty-one, just as the sun was beginning to set over the desert, I got my second wind. I crossed the finish line at thirty-nine hours in a respectable eleventh place. It was one of the most incredible feelings in my life—happiness, sadness, pain, euphoria, all wrapped into one. Adrenaline surged through every vein of my body. A feeling no drug could ever compare to.

Call me crazy, but Badwater was only preparation for my next big challenge: the Raid Gauloises. If you think that running through the desert is extreme, try a 520-mile race across one of the most treacherous mountain terrains in the world—the Himalayas. For eight days my team of five battled unbelievable obstacles. The worst of all was the air in Tibet. It was filled with yak dung. The stench was horrible and all the dust infected my lungs. As we gained altitude, my lungs began to fill with liquid, a life-threatening condition I later learned was called pulmonary edema. I felt faint, dizzy, and nauseated beyond belief. My body felt like it was turning against me and there was nothing I could do. At one point I honestly felt like I had reached the end of the road, that maybe I had pushed myself too hard, that maybe I would never be able to say good-bye to my mom and dad. This was as close to death as I had ever come.

A race doctor finally treated me with some very powerful medicine. It caused my lungs to vomit up fluid over the next six hours. To this day I don't know what she gave me, but I do know that it saved my life. Unbelievably, a few hours later I felt well enough to continue racing and finished with my teammates in only eight days.

Still recovering from that near-fatal lung infection, I had another challenge scheduled for the year 2000: the Grand Slam of Ultrarunning. It's actually four separate hundred-mile races called ultramarathons, run through some of the most difficult terrains in the United States. "Old Dominion"—one hundred miles through the Virginia Mountains, where I battled horseflies and blood-sucking ticks. "Western States"—a hundred miles through the Sierra Nevada Mountains of California, where I descended from freezing snowy peaks to scorching desert canyons. "Leadville"—a hundred miles through the Colorado Rockies, where at an altitude of twelve thousand feet I could hardly catch my breath. "Wasatch"—a hundred miles through the Utah mountains, where I climbed trails with over twenty-six thousand feet of elevation gain, like scaling the Empire State Building twenty-one times.

What does not kill me makes me stronger! Those words made me think there must be another challenge waiting to be conquered. I had survived the unbelievable, extreme heat of Badwater and the treacherous, rugged terrain of the Himalayan Mountains, four ultramarathons across the United States, now what? I needed something else to finish off this incredible year.

Could there be something else? Yes, there was. One night while watching television I just happened to catch the *Guinness World Records* show. A feature on the "24-Hour Physical Fitness Challenge," what's been dubbed "the World's Fittest Man" competition, caught my attention. Now, that was a challenge. It consisted of thirteen varied fitness events performed over a twenty-four-hour time period. I had done one or even two different events in one race, but never thirteen. The next day I wrote to Guinness World Records to find out how to apply and geared up for the challenge.

I was a good runner and biker, but some of my other events needed work. After brushing up on my swimming, kayaking, rowing, and NordicTrack, I felt ready to start. One cold Friday night in December, while most people were out on dates at the movies or home with their families by the fireplace, I was about to attempt a fitness world record. Thankfully, many of my friends and clients came out to support and cheer me on.

First the bike. One hundred miles circling around a quarter-mile running track; that's four hundred laps. (Guinness World Records required that I use a running track so that measurements could be recorded exactly.) Then on to running, hiking, and power walking. Combined I did the equivalent of a marathon. That was another hundred laps around the track. After twelve hours at the track the sun finally started to rise. Next, I raced to a nearby canal to complete six miles of kayaking. There, I started to get my second wind. Maybe I really could break the world record. Next, a two-mile swim in the pool. Luckily it was indoors, otherwise my body would have frozen. Then to the gym—ten miles on the NordicTrack cross-country ski machine, and another ten on the rowing machine. I was really flying through the events now. Only five more events, but these were the real tough ones. Talk about an intense calisthenics workout, worse than anything in that military "fat-boy program." I knew I had to kick some butt now if I wanted to break that record. Three thousand crunches, eleven hundred push-ups, eleven hundred leg lifts, and eleven hundred jumping jacks. To top it off I lifted a total of 278,540 pounds on ten different weight-lifting machines. My muscles ached for a couple days after that.

I notified *Guinness World Records*. Three months later it was official, I had broken the "24-Hour Physical Fitness Challenge" world record. In no time my amazing achievement had made national and international headlines. The media had proclaimed me "the World's Fittest Man." (Not just for breaking the Guinness World Record, but for all the other extreme challenges I completed that year.)

So that's how I became "the World's Fittest Man." I'm telling you about this journey not because I want to brag about all of my achievements and not because I'm special or different; I'm telling you this so you can see what's humanly possible. And what's achievable is different for everyone. My hundred laps around the track probably sounds like a lot. So does swimming two miles. All of that is relative. For you, the equivalent may be finishing your first 5K race or swimming a few laps in the pool without getting out of breath.

Most important, I'm telling you this so you can see that it really is possible to change your life around. That you can overcome seemingly insurmountable obstacles—obesity, addiction, and depression—like I did. The only obstacles are the ones you create for yourself. Most important, I'm telling you this because I'm just like you. That if I did it, so can you. Read on and I'll show you how to change your life and how to become "the World's Fittest You."

MY PROMISE

'm sure you've heard and seen lots of promises about losing weight and getting in shape. I hear them too. Some pills promise you'll lose twenty pounds without exercising. Some exercise plans promise a perfect body without really breaking a sweat.

My promise to you is simple: I did it, so can you. I lost the weight. I got in shape. I turned my life around. By following my program I promise that you can too.

I can't promise that you'll look like a model and have the perfect body after four weeks. I don't think anyone can make that promise. What I can promise is that you will see and feel changes in your body—and life—after four weeks. Those changes will be different for each of you reading my book and following my program. But I guarantee you will see changes and results.

SEVEN SIMPLE PROMISES TO YOU

I encourage you to take a picture of yourself at the beginning of the program and file it away. Then at the end of the four weeks take another one and see how your body has changed, not just on the outside but on the inside. By the end of my four-week program you will:

- get stronger, healthier, and leaner by making small, simple changes in your life
- discover the tools and means for a life of fitness
- achieve a positive approach to eating without dieting
- challenge yourself to reach new fitness limits
- look at your reflection and be happy with the person looking back at you
- make "fitness" fun so you continue building a better body
- develop an individualized program for achieving your personal fitness goals

My first promise, that you'll live a healthier and happier life, is really one of the most important. Sure, you want to look great, but you can't do anything without a body that is healthy and lean from the inside out. And I also promise that you will be able to do it all by making small, simple changes. Yes, you will have to put in the time and the effort. As I'll show you later on, there's no magic pill or gadget that's going to get you healthier. It's all up to you. But I'll be there every step of the way as you make all of these small changes. For instance, I'll show you how to gradually make small substitutions in your diet and to gradually cut out harmful saturated fats. Like for breakfast I used to smear loads of butter on white bread toast. I grew up doing that. By substituting a nutritious whole-grain bread and some farm-fresh jam or jelly, you can cut out lots of calories and fat while at the same time adding fiber to keep you feeling full. That's what I mean by a small change.

As a personal trainer I've helped hundreds of people get in shape. What I always tell my clients is that you can give a man a fish for a day or teach him how to fish for a lifetime. I know it sounds simple—maybe too simple—but, believe me, I have found it to be so true. What I promise you'll get from this book and my program are the tools "to fish for a lifetime." First, I'll get you started on a day-by-day, four-week program called "Shock Your Body." What's so unique about my program is that it will give you the means to get fitter and healthier for your entire lifetime. So many weight-loss and fitness programs don't work for people because—as you probably know yourself—it's just about a quick fix. Lose those twenty pounds over the weekend or get those rock-solid abs without doing a crunch. In Chapter 9, "Fit, Fitter, Fittest," I'll show you how to transition from my four-week program to an entire lifetime of fitness.

If you're like me, you've probably tried all those crazy fad dieting gimmicks. Take it from me, they simply don't work. Yes, I've lost weight on those diets, but no sooner did I lose the weight than it came right back. So what I promise to you is that you won't be dieting at all on my program. And I promise that I'll hardly even use that word. What you'll achieve through my unique ten-step "Power of Positive Eating" program is a healthful way to eat and look at food. I don't want you to see food as horrible or evil. It's not. You need food to live a healthy and happy life. Once I show you how to change your relationship with food so that it's a positive force in your life, you'll never have to think about dieting again.

My own greatest personal challenge was breaking the Guinness World Record. As I told you, that fitness challenge really took me to a new level of fitness and continues to keep me motivated to work out. It's like a job. If you don't have a challenge for yourself at work, you'll probably get bored and won't perform well at whatever job you do. Now, a challenge doesn't have to be a crazy fitness competition like the one I did; it can be something simple and fun you can do with your friends and family: a 5K Fun Run or an AIDS Walk. In my "Challenge Yourself!" chapter I'll help you find a challenge that's right for your fitness level. Most of all, a fitness challenge will keep you motivated to continue your lifelong goal of a healthy and fit life.

So much of our society is based on looking good. We're inundated with images of beautiful people and bodies. Just look at the cover of those men's magazines and you'll surely see a guy with rock-solid, six-pack abs. And open up a women's magazine and you'll see models so thin they defy an actual dress size. But living a healthy and happy life is so much more than just looking good. A lot of models and celebrities may look great on the outside, but on the inside they're a mess.

Just look at all the headlines about celebrities addicted to drugs and getting into all sorts of trouble. You'd think they'd have it easy. What this tells you is that it's not just about looking great in the mirror. It's so important to ultimately be happy with who's looking back at you in that very same mirror.

I can't tell you how many of my clients come to me saying how they're so bored with going to the gym and how their workouts have become stagnant. In fact, that's probably the biggest complaint I get from new clients, that they've stopped working out because it's so darn boring. So many people do the same workout day after day. Believe it or not, it's probably the same workout they've been doing since high school. Then, they tell me they're not seeing any results. Of course not! Your body adapts to that workout and stays at the exact same level. It's like going to the movies every weekend and seeing the exact same movie. How boring is that?

Your body is an amazing piece of machinery. You'd be surprised, it can take just about anything that you do. When it comes to working out, you've got to have a lot of variety, a lot of variation, because your body adapts so quickly. If you do the same thing over and over, believe me, nothing is going to change. I promise to show you how to add variety with a unique tool I call the FIT Equation. I guarantee that this equation will add variety and fun to your workouts. That's right, I'm going to make sure that you have "fitness" fun. I know to many of you that sounds like a contradiction in terms. How can you have fun working out? You'll see—by the end of my "Shock Your Body" program, I promise that you won't be dreading that next workout. Whether you're at home or at the gym, I'll show you simple ways to spice up your workouts and push your body so that you'll keep getting stronger and leaner.

JOE, WHAT'S YOUR SECRET?

When I broke the Guinness World Record I can't tell you how many people kept asking me questions about getting fit. How did you do it?

How did you get in such great shape? How did you do all those crunches and push-ups? I remember a television interviewer asking me, "What's your secret? Is it in your genes? Are you preprogrammed to be fit?" Of course not. My genes are no better than anyone else's. The secret is there is no secret. There is no magic bullet. There is no quick fix. There is no eight-minutes-to-get-fit program. What it's about is hard work and making the promise and commitment to yourself to change. If you've done that, you're halfway there. The next half is my job. I'll show you how to get the results you want.

So many people believe that to lose weight you have to enroll in an expensive program, buy lots of special food and supplements, or follow the regimen of a fad-diet guru. But that's not true. Research shows that most successful weight losers actually do it on their own.

HOW I DID IT

I developed this program through years of working with people like you as part of my personal training company. I've helped housewives, executives, mothers, fathers, and even children get in shape. I've also gone to corporations and helped busy people like you find the time, energy, and motivation to become fit. Through all these people's sweat and my own training for competitions like the Guinness challenge, I know what works and what doesn't. I know that if you want to become the World's Fittest You you're going to have to work. So memorize these words: YOU WILL HAVE TO WORK. You're going to have to work at changing the way you eat, the way you move, and the way you think. This is about making a commitment to improving your life. In the end you truly appreciate and value things more when you make that commitment.

SMALL CHANGES . . . BIG RESULTS

Whether you're new to working out or want to take your body to the next level, you've got to have a plan. What's so great about "the

World's Fittest You" is that this book is really about YOU! No matter what your level of fitness. I'll show you how to develop an individualized program that will work for you. It's also important to have goals to keep you on track, motivated, and focused. In Chapter 2, "Getting Started," I'll help you assess your fitness level and goals. Then, in the rest of the book, I'll show you how you can tailor my program to your specific needs.

Think about all the times you've tried to make changes in your life. You wanted to change careers. You wanted to get married. You wanted to have a family. You wanted more success. You'll remember that these changes didn't come overnight. They didn't even happen in a week or two. Instead, these changes happened slowly, in small steps. I remember that first ten-speed bike I wanted. It cost $50. At the time, $50 was a lot to me. So to get that bike I baled hay for my grandpa and did odd jobs for other farmers. After weeks and weeks of working hard, scrimping and saving, I got a bike. Making lifestyle changes, the way you eat and work out, is no different. The effort you put in now will pay off later.

So the core of my book, my program, is about how to make these small changes. And how these small changes will have big results for you. By *big* I mean results that match your specific goals and are, above all, realistic and achievable.

I'M HERE FOR YOU

My final promise is that I'm going to be here for you. As you read through the book and try out the different meal plans and workout techniques, you're bound to have questions. That's part of the process. You have to ask questions. So jot those questions down and send them off to me. You can contact me anytime through my Web site; there's a special area for sending me your questions. Even if you don't have a question and just want to give me an update about your successes, that's great too. You can also access more information and get helpful tips on my Web site.

GETTING STARTED: BECOMING THE WORLD'S FITTEST YOU

CHAPTER 2

I DID IT. . . . SO CAN YOU

There is a reason I call this section of the book "Becoming the World's Fittest You." No matter what your shape, size, or fitness level . . . this program is designed for you. It worked for me because I was ready for change. Sometimes change can be scary, if you're not sure what you want in life. I was there, too, when I found myself wandering the country after leaving the military. Did I want to go back to college? Did I want to be a lawyer? Did I want to get married and have kids? Instead of looking inside myself and seeing where I wanted to be in life, I let bad habits and lack of self-control take over.

You've picked up this book and read my story; that's a start. You've obviously decided you want to get your body into shape. That's an even better start. Beginning a new way of life, getting a healthy lifestyle, is the hardest part. Just admitting to yourself that you're ready for change is difficult enough. So I congratulate you on this very first step!

Now that you've made that first step, and seen how I turned my own life around, it's your turn. What follows is a step-by-step program that changed my life and can change yours too. You'll see later on that what makes my program so unique is that by simply making small changes, you'll be getting big results. You'll be shaping up, eating smart, and feeling great. . . . It's about becoming "the World's Fittest You." It's a blueprint for change that won't leave you feeling like you're missing out on all the things you like in life. Remember: It's all about YOU. That's why my program is different. It's not about a diet, or a specific set of exercises, it's about you and changing your lifestyle. It's about you taking control.

If you're looking for quick fixes and crazy promises, I'm sorry to say you're not going to find them here. Ultimately, you're going to have to work for it. But with me as your coach and personal advisor, you'll have lots of help along the way. Just think how proud you will feel when you have accomplished your goals through your own hard work. The journey of ten thousand miles begins with one step. So, let's take that first step.

Throughout this chapter I've included tools and charts that will help you keep track of your thoughts and progress throughout your "World's Fittest You" program. This section will help you get started and on your way to becoming "the World's Fittest You."

THE "WORLD'S FITTEST YOU" PROGRAM IS FOR YOU

So what is "the World's Fittest You," anyway? First of all it's different for everyone. Maybe you've never done any exercise and want to start moving and feeling better about yourself. Maybe you want to lose those last ten pounds that you've been trying to get rid of for years. Maybe you've tried lots of "fad" diets and want to lose weight permanently this time. Or maybe you're in good shape already but want that breakthrough to the next level of fitness. Whatever shape or size you are now, this program is for you because you can design it to meet your needs.

Later on you'll see there will be many ways you can adapt my program to your own goals. In order to make changes in the way you look and feel, you'll have to modify the way you eat and move. You'll see that the "Power of Positive Eating" program will have lots of choices, options, strategies, and tips. Over four weeks I'll help you reduce the "bad" or saturated fat in your diet and replace it with "good fats," healthy whole grains, fruits, and vegetables. By doing this you'll be cutting back on excess calories. That's really the key. Then, following my "Shock Your Body" program, you'll choose activities that are fun and fit your particular lifestyle. I'll show you how to gradually add new activities and how to change things up with my breakthrough FIT Equation. All of this will transform your body with amazing results. Just wait and see.

TAKING INVENTORY

Stop for a minute. At this point you're going to take inventory of your life. By *inventory* I mean just make a list of what your life is like now. Where are you now? Are you healthy? Are you happy with the way you look and feel? Are you satisfied with what you see when you look in the mirror? Are you happy with your job? Your professional life? Do you have friends and family you can talk to?

I remember, when I was at my lowest point living in New Orleans, I looked at where I was and what I was doing. You'll remember from my story that my life was falling apart. Well, I took inventory. I realized I wasn't happy with my job. I wasn't happy with the way I looked and felt. All the eating and drinking made me feel awful about myself. But before I could make any changes, I had to take inventory. Maybe I didn't know it at the time, but that's what I was doing—taking inventory. Once I did that I knew I wanted to change, not just what I ate, but my whole lifestyle.

MEDICAL INVENTORY

Before starting any exercise and fitness program you should check with your doctor. It's important that he or she give you the okay to start. On your visit you'll also want some other medical information as part of your "Getting Started" inventory. Record this information in the chart on page 12 so you can use it for future comparison.

BLOOD PRESSURE

Blood pressure measures the strength with which your heart pumps blood through your body. The pressure itself is determined by the force and amount of blood pumped as well as the size of your arteries. If you have high blood pressure, called hypertension, you're at a higher risk for developing a heart attack, heart failure, stroke, and kidney failure. The American Heart Association considers 120/80 or below a desirable level.

Becoming the World's Fittest You can help lower your blood pressure.

CHOLESTEROL

Cholesterol is a normal substance in your body. It's found in your bloodstream and all your body's cells. But when you have too much cholesterol, it causes heart disease and puts you at risk for heart attacks. Ask your doctor to perform a complete cholesterol test that includes HDL, LDL, and triglycerides.

You get cholesterol in two basic ways. Your body makes some, but most of it comes from eating animal products that contain saturated fats. I'll get into this more later, but the bottom line is that you can help control the level of cholesterol in your blood by changing the way you eat. The general recommendation is to keep your total cholesterol below 200. Reducing the amount of saturated fat in your diet is one way to control your cholesterol levels. Your doctor may also prescribe cholesterol-lowering drugs.

There are two types of cholesterol that you need to know about. LDL (low-density lipoprotein) is known as "bad" cholesterol. When there's too much LDL in your blood, it builds up and clogs your arteries, causing a heart attack or stroke. A desirable level of LDL is under 100, but near optimal is 100–129.

HDL (high-density lipoprotein) is known as "good" cholesterol. A high level of HDL can actually protect against heart disease. While LDL accumulates in your arteries, it's believed that HDL can remove some of this buildup. In this way HDL acts as a sort of street sweeper in your arteries, removing plaque buildup and "sweeping" it out of your body. The more HDL, the better; a desirable level is 60, but anything over 40 is good.

Triglycerides are just beginning to be recognized as important to monitor. Like cholesterol they are used to move fatty acids through the bloodstream. Drinking a lot of alcohol and eating white sugar can significantly raise your triglyceride level. High levels of triglycerides are now understood to put you at risk for heart disease too. Generally speaking, a triglyceride level under 150 is desirable.

Becoming the World's Fittest You can help lower your total cholesterol, LDL (bad cholesterol), and triglycerides.

Becoming the World's Fittest You can help raise your HDL (good cholesterol).

BLOOD SUGAR READING

A blood-sugar or glucose test performed by your doctor measures the amount of sugar in your blood. When you eat a high-sugar-content food like a candy bar or cookie, your level of blood sugar increases. The hormone insulin, however, regulates that amount. Diabetes, the sixth leading killer among diseases in the United States, occurs when your body doesn't produce enough insulin. There are two types of diabetes. Type 1 is diagnosed during childhood and is thought to be genetic or inherited. Type 2 diabetes, often referred to as adult-onset diabetes, is closely related to overeating, obesity, and lack of physical activity. If your blood sugar levels are too high, that puts you at risk for type 2 diabetes. A normal reading is 70 to 110 after eight hours of not eating.

Becoming the World's Fittest You can reduce your risk of developing type 2 diabetes.

RESTING HEART RATE

This test measures the number of times your heart beats per minute when you're not exercising or doing any physical activity. It's a very good indicator of your overall fitness level. If you're in good shape, your resting heart rate will most likely be low, and means that your heart is doing less work to pump blood through your body. If you haven't been working out in a while, you'll probably have a higher resting heart rate. A desirable resting heart rate is between sixty and ninety beats per minute.

Becoming the World's Fittest You can help lower your resting heart rate.

BMI

BMI or Body Mass Index is a measurement of your total body fat based on your height and weight. It's a more accurate reflection of your total body fat than looking at just your weight. A healthy range is from 18.5 to 24.9. You can figure this out at home by plugging your height and weight into the BMI calculator on my Web site.

Becoming the World's Fittest You can help lower your body mass index.

MEDICAL INVENTORY CHART

Test	Date: _____
Blood pressure	
Total cholesterol	
LDL	
Triglycerides	
HDL	
Blood sugar reading	
Resting heart rate	
BMI	

PHYSICAL-FITNESS TESTS

Now that you've recorded your medical starting point, you're going to need to perform a quick physical-fitness inventory. If you've done fitness activities before, then these tests will probably seem easy. That's okay. Do them anyway so you can see your progress. If you're new to fitness, then these tests might be more challenging. Don't be disappointed with your results. There's no pass or fail. No one is going to be grading you. These are for measuring your own assessment. Since my "Shock Your Body" program is about total fitness, you'll be working your entire body in three different ways: flexibility, strength, and cardiovascular or cardio endurance.

The Flexibility Test

This test measures how limber your body is, how easy it is to move your body through a wide range of motions.

Place a yardstick on the floor and tape it down at the fifteen-inch mark. Warm up your body a little by walking around the block or up and down a flight of stairs. Sit on the floor with the yardstick between your legs a little wider than hip width apart. Make sure the "0" is closest to your body. Place one hand on top of the other and slowly stretch forward with your fingertips on the yardstick. The farther your reach, the higher your score. Do the test three times and record your highest score, rounding off to the nearest inch.

The Strength Tests

These two tests measure the strength of your upper body and abdominal muscles. Muscular strength is important because it helps you build a leaner and more toned body. It also helps you control your weight, since muscle tissue burns more calories than fat.

Push-up Test

Take a look at page 214 to see how to perform a push-up using proper form. Even if you think you know how to do a push-up—I'm sure you've probably done them in high school—look at my demonstration photos and practice a few times. If you're really having trouble doing a regular push-up, do the modified variation. I usually recommend that beginners, or people who have not worked out in a while, stick to the modified variation. Do as many push-ups as you can without a break. When you can't do anymore that's your fitness level. Record the number.

Crunch Test

Take a look at page 242 of this book to see how to do a crunch. Do as many crunches as you can in sixty seconds. Make sure to keep your chin off your chest and use your abdominal muscles, not your shoulders. Record the number.

Endurance Test

Cardio endurance indicates how well your lungs, heart, and blood vessels deliver oxygen to the rest of your body. Cardio is an important part of the program because it helps burn calories and thereby controls your weight. It also improves your cardiovascular system, to help prevent coronary heart disease. Remember, your heart is the most important muscle in your body, not your biceps.

Find an eight-inch-high stair or bench. Step up with your right foot, then your left foot. Step down with your right foot, then your left. You might want to say, "Up, up, down, down," to help you keep a steady pace. Practice this a few times before you start the test. When you're comfortable with the movement, time yourself for three minutes. As soon as you stop, take your pulse. Record your pulse rate.

PHYSICAL FITNESS INVENTORY

Test	Date: _____
Flexibility	
Push-up	
Crunch	
Cardio Endurance	

ARE YOU A POWER POSITIVE EATER?

Now I want you to take inventory of what you eat. Becoming "the World's Fittest You" is more than just working out. It's changing the way you eat and think about food. I call my eating program the "Power of Positive Eating" because it's really about eating, not dieting (more about this in Chapter 4). To get a better picture of your eating habits now, let's see if you are a Power Positive Eater. After you complete my program, you can take inventory again and see how your eating habits have changed.

Do I eat three small meals and three snacks per day?   Yes   No

Do I notice the size of my portions?   Yes   No

Do I drink six to eight glasses of water per day?   Yes   No

Do I read the food label before I buy food?   Yes   No

Do I know what food is in my refrigerator
and where it's located?   Yes   No

Do I substitute mustard or salsa for mayonnaise?   Yes   No

Do I keep track of what I eat and how I feel
when I am eating?   Yes   No

Do I tell the waiter exactly how I want my food
prepared when I go out for meals?   Yes   No

Do I plan what I'm going to eat for the next few days?   Yes   No

Do I reward myself for my healthy eating habits?   Yes   No

How did you do? If you answered yes for eight to ten of these questions you're already on the right track. If not, that's okay. The "Power of Positive Eating" plan in Chapter 4 will help you change that.

DEFINING "THE WORLD'S FITTEST YOU"

Now that you've taken inventory on your life, where you are at this very moment, it's time to set some goals. This is really important, otherwise you won't be able to see your progress and this will diminish your motivation. So what's a goal? For me a goal is something I want to achieve and to which I can see the end point. When I failed that military fitness test, I was devastated and embarrassed. At that stage my goal was to get in shape, lose forty pounds, and kick butt on the test.

Maybe you don't need to pass a physical fitness test like I did, but you want to look and feel better. That's a goal. But remember it has to be realistic and have a set end point. If you've never really done any fitness activities before, then maybe your goal is just to do a fitness activity at least five or six times a week for a period of four weeks. I know that may sound like a lot at first, but you'll see—once you start you'll want to do even more. If you want to lose inches off your waist, set a number and time period. Be specific. Don't just say, "I want to look like Cindy Crawford." That kind of standard is probably unrealistic. When I first started changing my lifestyle, my goal certainly wasn't to become the World's Fittest Man. Heck, I could barely even run a mile. Set your goal as it pertains to you individually. For instance, set your goal as maybe one inch off your waist in four weeks, one pound each week, work out every day, or tone up your abs. For you fitness buffs, maybe your goal is to increase your upper-body strength and tone up your abs or even run a marathon. Whatever your goals are, jot them down here and be specific:

WORLD'S FITTEST YOU GOALS

1. _____
2. _____
3. _____
4. _____

A PLAN OF ACTION!

When I was training for the Badwater Ultramarathon, that 135-mile trek across Death Valley, California, I definitely had a plan. I started off each day with a 7–10-mile run on a treadmill in a special room that could heat up to 140 degrees. And on the weekends I would run anywhere up to 50 miles at a time. I know this definitely sounds extreme, but I stuck to my plan and have now finished Badwater twice.

You've set your goals and now you're going to need a plan to achieve them. By following the program in Chapters 5–8 you have a plan. These chapters will take you through a day-by-day, week-by-week program to change your lifestyle so you're eating better and moving your body more. You'll see that the plans are based on my own training program. It's how I got to be "the World's Fittest Man," so I know it can help you too. This applies to even the most simple, basic goals.

MONITOR, CHECK IN, AND REWARD!

It's important that you set checkpoints. I like to monitor myself every week when I'm training for an event. That way I know how far I've come and how much more training I need. When I was training for the Guinness World Records fitness competition, I checked myself about every day. I would increase my pounds lifted, add fifty more push-ups, or add an extra couple miles to my weekly total. I would reach a checkpoint and then set the bar a little higher. I know that must sound like a lot, but I worked slowly up to that point.

If your goal is to lose weight, then you might want to weigh yourself every week at the same time of day so you get a consistent weight. If your goal is just to start an activity program, then check in with yourself at the end of the week. Did I work out five or six times this week? These checkpoints really keep you on track and motivated. They helped me tremendously and I know they can help you too. Consistency is definitely the key. Record keeping and logs are there to show progress or the need for change. Studies have shown that those people who keep track of what they eat and how much they work out have better results. And the more details the better. In fact, one study found that those who kept a detailed diary of each and every workout lost twice as much weight as those who didn't.

And finally, when you've made it to the checkpoint and you're on track with your goal, reward yourself. Don't make it food, because you'll see that in the "Power of Positive Eating" program you already have a food reward day. Instead, make it something special, something you wouldn't normally do or buy. Research from the Cooper Institute shows that people who reward themselves are two to three times more likely to meet their physical activity goals than people who don't.

I'm a pretty simple guy, so I don't believe your rewards have to be anything expensive or extravagant. Here are some of the ways I reward myself:

- a new piece of outdoor gear
- extra time to read a book—the classics are my favorite
- a trip to the movies and a small popcorn
- a new pair of running shoes
- and my favorite, a good bottle of wine and a great cigar

At the end of each week check in with yourself to record your progress:

World's Fittest You Checkpoints

	Week 1	Week 2	Week 3	Week 4
Goal 1				
Goal 2				
Goal 3				
Goal 4				

PICKING YOUR TEAM

When I decided to overcome my alcohol and eating problems, I know I couldn't have done it without the support of my mom and dad. They were there every step of the way, providing me with incredible motivation and just some old-fashioned parental love.

Whether it's e-mail or voice mail, establish a "World's Fittest You" team of family and friends. Make a list of three or four people with whom you'd like to share your successes. Write their names down next to your telephone and if you have a computer add them to your e-mail "buddy list." Whenever you reach a checkpoint, let them know. I know this may sound silly, but it really does help.

You might want to find a buddy and do the program together. Studies really show that working out with a friend can help you stick to your fitness and weight-loss program. The trick is finding someone who's more committed than you, that way if you slack off, your buddy will keep you going. If you know someone out there cares about your success, like my mom and dad did when I was struggling, you're more likely to stick with the program.

And if you have a setback, let your buddies know too. If these are people you really care about, I'm sure they'll give you words of encouragement. Most of my friends and family like to support me even when I'm feeling down. If you give these people the opportunity to help you keep toward your goals, they will.

WORLD'S FITTEST YOU BUDDY LIST

Buddy's Name	Phone	E-mail

HAVE "FITNESS FUN"!

I can't emphasize enough the importance of *fun*. So I'll say it again. Have fun! My own clients tell me that the main reason they stick with my program is because they love the variety. And you thought it was my charming personality. In my "Shock Your Body" program you'll see that there are lots of choices to keep you active, from walking to rowing. What's more, every Saturday of the program I've included a fun-filled workout that will get you out of the gym or house. So, whatever activity you choose, make it fun.

Some people ask me why I continue doing all these events and competitions. Sure, I love the challenge and excitement of a race. But more than that, it's just downright fun. It may not look like fun when I'm out there sweating and puffing away, but deep down I'm having the best time of my life. In the last chapter, "Challenge Yourself!," I've included lots of ways you can add fitness challenges to your program, whether it's a Breast Cancer Walk or a half marathon or maybe even something more extreme, like an adventure race, for you adrenaline junkies.

THE FIT EQUATION

CHAPTER 3

CHANGE IT UP

I hate using the word *exercise*. Although you'll see the word used a few times in this book, I like to refer to exercises as activities. *Exercises* makes you think of something you don't want to do. That's why you'll see my program is completely different. It's not about exercising at all, it's about activities, things you'll want to do, things that are fun, and won't take up lots of your time. If you're one of those people who get bored with exercise, you're not alone. Most Americans stop working out, not because they don't have time, commitment, or motivation but because of sheer monotony. That's right, boredom, some say, is the number-one reason people don't stick with a fitness program.

You'll see that my "Shock Your Body" program is about changing your fitness activities often so that you don't get bored. You'll actually get better results this way too. If you're doing the same routine day in and day out, week after week, your body will get accustomed to whatever you're doing to build muscle and lose weight. After a while those same routines won't be as effective and you'll either reach a plateau or stop altogether.

When I was getting ready for the "24-Hour Physical Fitness Challenge," I told you about earlier, I was training for thirteen separate events. Every day I was doing something completely different. One day I was in the pool swimming laps. The next day I was lifting weights in the gym. Then I was out there hiking and power walking. I got to be the World's Fittest Man because I was always challenging my body with something new. My body never knew what was coming.

Working out has to be fun so you keep moving and burning off those calories—and transforming that flab into well-toned muscle. Don't worry, I won't be asking you to train for a thirteen-event competition. But what I will be asking you to do is to make a commitment to make small changes in the way you move your body. We'll start off slowly and I'll show you how, by just making small changes with constant variation, you can have amazing results. A lot of the programs you may have tried didn't work for you because you're doing the same thing day in and day out. Boredom sets in and you just stop working out. All that is about to change.

WORLD'S FITTEST MAN'S FITNESS MYTH BUSTERS

Before we go any farther, I'd like to clear up some misconceptions. Over the years, as a personal trainer teaching both individuals and groups, I've really heard some crazy ideas about fitness and what people think does and doesn't work. Now I'd like to give it to you straight and dispel some of those fitness myths.

Fitness Myth

You can target certain problem spots like abs and love handles.

Fittest Man's Fitness Fact

I'd have to say, the two most frequently asked questions I get from my clients are "How do I get six-pack abs?" and "How do I get rid of these love handles?" Let me give it to you straight: Forget the idea of transforming a certain spot of your body. It just doesn't work. You can't simply tone one part of your body without working the entire body. Getting back to abs, there's a layer of fat, like a sweater, covering those muscles. Once you start cutting the fat and calories, once you start burning off calories through working out, and once you start strengthening and toning the muscles in your entire body, then you may start to see those six-pack abs—like pulling off that sweater. I can't guarantee it, but I can guarantee that you won't see those six-pack abs by just doing thousands of abdominal crunches each day. Results come from a well-rounded plan.

Fitness Myth

You can get fit with just eight minutes of physical activity a day.

Fittest Man's Fitness Fact

When you hear these kinds of claims, be wary. Eight minutes a day might be good for someone who has never exercised in his/her life before, but it's not enough for anyone seriously wanting to lose weight, get fit, and lead a healthy life. While there's much debate on exactly how much physical activity you need, there are proven standards. With my program you'll need to devote between thirty and sixty minutes per day, five to six days per week. I know that may sound like a lot, but if you really do want to become "the World's Fittest You," you are definitely going to have to work for it. There's no getting around that. What I'll promise is that if you are going to spend the time, I'll make sure you get the results you want and keep it fun and motivating.

Fitness Myth

Women who lift weights risk growing muscles like a man.

Fittest Man's Fitness Fact

For some reason women think that lifting weights will give them big bulging muscles like a man. The truth is that women and men develop muscles differently. Men have hormones that allow their bodies to bulk up. Women don't have those same hormones. Without the male hormone you won't get big and bulky. But you will get leaner and sexier.

Fitness Myth

You won't see results without feeling pain.

Fittest Man's Fitness Fact

My program is about "Shocking Your Body"—not causing pain. It's about working hard and getting results. So anyone who tells you that you have to torture your body and feel pain in order to get results is flat-out wrong. If at any point during my program you start to feel pain, then you should stop whatever you're doing and go see your doctor. Pain is usually a sign that you've injured something, not that you're getting better results. I always say, on the other side of pain is injury. Make sure to listen to your body.

Fitness Myth

You should always work out on an empty stomach.

Fittest Man's Fitness Fact

I always recommend having a little bit of food before you start your workout. Now, I'm not talking about a full meal, just a little snack to keep your blood sugar levels up throughout your workout. Even in the morning you should have a little something before you start your activities. You'll see on my "Power of Positive Eating" plan you'll be eating three snacks each day. I would suggest planning to have one of these snacks about thirty to forty-five minutes before your workout. You need the fuel to get you through a great workout.

Fitness Myth

You burn more calories if you exercise longer at lower and slower intensity.

Fittest Man's Fitness Fact

If your primary goal is weight loss, then the most important thing to remember is the total number of calories you've burned during the activity, not the percentage of calories coming from fat. A calorie is a calorie is a calorie no matter where it comes from. The harder your intensity, the more calories you burn, the more weight you can lose. It's that simple.

Fitness Myth

You need to take expensive muscle-building supplements and shakes to build a better body.

Fittest Man's Fitness Fact

When people see my body, they think I've gotten this way by taking some special muscle-building supplements or pills. Here's what I tell them: It's hard work and commitment that got me to where I am today, nothing else. Well, maybe a few pizzas too. Some programs you may have heard about require that you buy expensive bodybuilding supplements and special protein shakes to supplement your diet. If you follow my "Power of Positive Eating" plan, you'll be getting all the protein and just about all the minerals and vitamins you'll need. Save your money. These shakes and supplements are neither cheap nor necessary.

SHOCKING YOUR BODY INTO SHAPE

My "Shock Your Body" program incorporates a revolutionary new way of structuring your workout so that you get maximum results without having to spend hours and hours in the gym. It's called the FIT Equation. It's not a gimmick or a quick fix, but a technique of changing up your routine as frequently as possible to fight off what I call "Exercise Boredom."

The FIT Equation incorporates some of the latest exercise research from the American College of Sports Medicine (ACSM), one of the leading fitness research groups in the country. The ACSM sets many of the standards for how and how much to work out based on up-to-the-minute scientific research by the top exercise physiologists in the country. Some of their latest research involves a technique called nonlinear periodization. Simply put, nonlinear periodization involves the idea of changing your workout routine from day to day, with as much variation as possible. Research shows that varying your workout with such frequency not only relieves boredom, but can be more effective in reaching your fitness goals. I've taken some of this research about variation to help develop the FIT Equation.

All of this may sound complicated at first, creating lots of variation, but I'll show you how to do it step by step, day by day. Essentially, what you'll be doing is varying cardio and strength training in a total program that will "Shock Your Body" and muscles. Your body has a way of adapting very quickly to any fitness program that becomes routine. By doing the same thing over and over again, your body stays at the same level and doesn't get stronger. By "shocking" your muscles with different workout routines every day, you'll be keeping your body guessing. When I work with clients, sometimes I don't even tell them what they'll be doing that day. I'll surprise them with a different workout, something they're not accustomed to doing. After a while my clients actually like this way better, especially when they see results.

WHY TOTAL BODY?

You've probably heard about fitness programs that emphasize lifting weights over cardio. And others stress just cardio activities and no weight training at all. And some programs say you can buy "exercise in a bottle" and get fit by just popping a pill. As you'll see, my program works your total body—cardio activities to burn calories and strengthen your heart, strength-training activities to build muscle and tone your body, and stretching activities to lengthen your muscles and keep you limber. Remember, the key to weight loss is boosting your metabolism. The combination of strength training and cardio will give you a higher metabolic rate than just strength training alone.

WHAT IS THE FIT EQUATION?

So just how do you make working out fun and fight off "exercise boredom"? You'll see how it works in more detail in the actual four-week program starting in Chapter 5, but I'll first explain some of the basics and principles here to get you started. As I said, my unique formula to "Shock Your Body" is called the FIT Equation. The equation is made up of three variables: *Frequency*, *Intensity*, and *Time*. That's all you need to remember. It's that simple.

F FOR FREQUENCY

Frequency is the number of times you perform that activity, whether it's cardio, strength training, or flexibility. When you change the frequency, you'll be changing the number of times you're doing something. For cardio you'll see that the frequency is the number of times per week you do your activity, whether it's running, biking, or swimming. For strength training the frequency is the number of times you repeat a specific movement. It's very important that you mix up the frequency so that you're not doing the same routine every week.

I FOR INTENSITY

The intensity in the FIT Equation indicates how hard you'll be working. One of the biggest misunderstandings that I hear from my clients is that they feel like they have to work out at a hundred-percent effort every day. Don't get me wrong, I believe you have to work out hard to get results, but you sometimes might actually be working out too hard and therefore getting negative results. In some cases working out too hard can also lead to injury like repetitive stress to your muscles. By changing the Intensity variable you'll be getting the most from your workout. Some days you will be going hard, other days not so hard. Like everything else in your body your muscles, bones, and joints need to rest in order to grow stronger and leaner. So for each of the cardio and strength-training activities you'll be varying the intensity of the FIT Equation. Think of the intensity as a fire or flame burning inside of you. Some days that flame will be burning bright and the fire strong—igniting you to push your body to its limits. Other days that flame will be burning less intensely and therefore your effort will not be as strong. Again, variety is the key.

T FOR TIME

The last part of the FIT Equation is Time. While there is a minimum amount of time that you should be spending doing your fitness activities, the length won't be the same every day. For cardio activities the Time is the overall amount you'll be doing that activity. When you're first starting out, the Time you spend may be less than the minimum recommended. And I'll actually give you the option to divide the time up into two or three more manageable smaller workouts. You could be walking ten minutes around the block during your lunch break and then an extra ten minutes after work on your way to your car or train. Research shows that it doesn't really matter whether you do all your cardio at once or break it up into a few sessions, you can get the same benefit.

For your strength-training activities the Time variable will mean something a little different. Rather than the overall amount of time you spend lifting your weights, the Time will be the amount of time you rest in between activities. (You'll need a watch that shows seconds to keep track of this.)

THE THREE TYPES OF WORLD'S FITTEST YOU ACTIVITIES

1. Cardio

Cardiovascular or cardio activities are an important part of my program. The great thing about cardio activities is that you have so many different options to choose from. Whether you like to be indoors or out, there's something here for you. You just have to do it. Most of my clients like to choose a few activities—I say, the more the merrier. That way you won't get bored doing the same activity over and over again. At first you'll want to stick to an activity, like walking or bicycling, that you're familiar with. As you continue with the program, I encourage you to try new things. Before becoming "the World's Fittest Man" I had never tried kayaking, and never thought it would be an activity I would like. Now it's a part of my routine, and whenever I have the opportunity to take a kayak for a spin, I do it. Whatever activities you decide to choose, you'll get some of these benefits:

- Burn calories
- Decrease your body fat
- Reduce your risk of cardiovascular disease
- Decrease your fatigue
- Enhance your sense of well-being
- Boost your immune system
- Cleanse your body of toxins

Cardio and the FIT Equation

If you've ever done cardio activities before—and I'm sure most of you have at some point in your life—you've probably done the activity just to get it over with, without thinking too much about how or what you're doing. Maybe you just jogged a few miles at an even pace. That's great if you did, but now we're going to take that to a new level with the FIT Equation.

The first thing you need to know is that in order to get the benefits of cardio activities, you have to do it more than once a week. If you really want to become "the World's Fittest You," you're going to have to follow some fundamental standards based on scientific research. That research shows that you'll need to do cardio activities at least three to five times per week, for at least twenty to sixty minutes, at an intensity of 55 to 90 percent of your maximum heart rate.

With these standards as a guide, here's how the FIT Equation works. The Frequency is the number of times per week you'll do cardio activities. Most weeks it will be three or four. When I'm training for a big race like a marathon, I may just focus on that one cardio activity like running. If you're training for a race or event, you, too, might increase the frequency of your cardio workouts so that you can increase your endurance and speed for the event. Overall, I don't recommend doing more than five cardio workouts each week, especially if you're just doing the same activity. If you do, you really increase your risk of injury. I suggest mixing up the activities as much as you can so that you don't overuse the same muscles and risk injury.

Now on to Intensity. You can measure the intensity of your cardio activities many different ways. Some people like to use a heart rate monitor—obviously the faster your heart rate, the higher the intensity. I like to use a different method, one that's a little simpler and doesn't require any special equipment. It's called the Rate of Perceived Exertion (RPE). It works like this: Your workout intensity is rated on a scale of 1 through 10. An intensity of 1 is no activity. A 10 represents an all-out effort, like a sprint at the end of a race (see page 31). One way to help you decide on the number is to pay attention to how hard you're breathing and how hard your heart is pumping.

The Time variable will tell you two things. First, it tells you how long you'll be doing the cardio activity on a particular day of the program. Second, the Time variable also tells you how long you'll be working at a specific intensity. This is called "interval training" and it's really an important part of my program. Be prepared—if you choose a cardio outside, you're going to need a watch with a stopwatch feature.

In the gym you're covered, because most pieces of cardio equipment have a built-in stopwatch to monitor your time. Let's take a closer look at one of the cardio workouts that you'll find throughout the rest of the book to understand how the FIT Equation works.

RATE OF PERCEIVED EXERTION

1	Nothing
2	Very easy
3	Easy
4	Comfortable
5	Somewhat difficult
6	Difficult
7	Hard
8	Very hard
9	Extremely hard
10	Unbearable

This is a workout I did myself. I chose outdoor cycling. During this twenty-minute workout I varied my intensity according to the elapsed time. So for the first five minutes, which is my warm-up, I rode at an intensity of 2, just to get my blood flowing and my muscles into gear.

Activity	Frequency	Intensity	Time
Outdoor cycling	3 times per week	2	minutes 1–5
		5	minutes 6–10
		6	minutes 11–16
		2	minutes 17–20

Now, I'm up to minute six. Using the RPE chart as a guide, I increased my intensity to 5 for this interval: minutes six through ten. For the time interval eleven to sixteen I worked a little harder and increased my intensity a bit more to 6. Then, for the final interval, minutes seventeen to twenty, I slowed down to an intensity of 2. It's really important to let your body cool down and your heart rate slow down before ending your cardio workout.

Burning Calories with the FIT Equation

Remember, the formula for losing weight is simple. Increase the number of calories you expend with physical activity while at the same time decreasing the number of calories you take in. While you'll burn calories during your strength training, you'll burn lots more doing cardio activities. That doesn't mean you should only do cardio. Part of building a leaner, healthier body means building your muscles through strength training too. In the Cardio Activities I've listed in Appendix A, I've indicated the number of calories you'll burn for each activity. This is a very basic guide—and it all depends on how hard you work. The harder you work, the more calories you burn.

When to Do Your Cardio

If you want to burn off fat, then the best time to do your cardio workout is in the morning. Some studies show that when you do your cardio on an almost empty stomach—that's usually first thing in the morning—you enhance your fat burning during and after your workout. I suggest you have a little snack even in the morning. If you've just eaten a big meal, or have in the past six hours, your body is going to use the carbohydrates from your meal as fuel. However, if you work out on a relatively empty stomach, with just a small meal for energy, your body will go right for the fat cells to get fuel, optimizing your fat burning. Let's be clear: If the morning doesn't work for you, then anytime during the day is better than no time.

Choosing the "Fittest" Cardio Activities for You

How do you know which cardio activity is right for your body? First, know your body's limits. Some of my clients tell me right from the start that high-impact activities like running put too much stress on their leg muscles and joints. If that's the case, don't take part in them. It will just cause you injury and pain. In the end you won't stick with the program. Second, choose activities that match your personality. I enjoy the outdoors, so I choose activities like running and biking. I like the openness and sense of freedom. Even when I'm traveling to different cities, I'll find a park or bike path to use for my workouts. Other activities, like swimming back and forth in a pool, don't suit my personality as much. I swim, though, to change things up in my routine and give my legs a break. To find out your "cardio fitness personality," take this quick test to help choose your "fittest" activities. After you answer the questions, go through the Cardio Activities in Appendix A and pick five activities that match your personality.

CARDIO FITNESS PERSONALITY TEST

1. Do I like to work out indoors or outdoors?

You'll see that I've divided the cardio activities into two sections. First the gym activities that are indoors and then the outdoor activities. Some of my clients are very busy and like the convenience of going to the gym and not having to worry about weather conditions. They also say that using the exercise machines helps them control the speed and intensity of their workout better. Others really love the exhilaration of being outside. It's up to you.

2. Do I get bored quickly with cardio or do I like doing the same activity often?

Even if you like doing the same activity all the time, I'm going to encourage you to vary your activities as much as possible. That's why I've included such a comprehensive list of activities—to show you that there's so much out there to try. But if you do get bored quickly, you might try doing two or three different machines in one workout. Start out on the bicycle, then switch to the treadmill, and then finish up on the elliptical trainer.

3. Do I like activities alone or do I like the motivation of a group?

I really enjoy the solitude of going for a run or bike ride by myself. It gives me time to think and enjoy some peace and get away from stresses of the day. Some of my clients really like the motivation of group activities. In the boot-camp-style workout classes I teach, the men and women push each other along. If you like that kind of workout then try a spinning class or join a local running club.

4. Do I like activities where I have to learn a new skill?

Most of the cardio activities in the program are very basic and don't require that you have any special skills. The basic goal, as I've said before, is just to get out there and do something. But if you decide to pick an activity like in-line skating and you've never done it before, then be prepared to learn the skills to do it. I've rated each activity for skill level, so choose wisely. Pick one that matches your skill level.

5. Am I prone to injury or have I injured myself in the past?

The point of doing these activities is to get in great shape and have fun. The last thing I want is for you to get injured. When choosing your activities, be aware of the injury risk level. If you know that your knees can't take the stress of pounding pavement, then stick to the activities that have a low impact level. I know it sounds like common sense, but I've had many clients come to me who don't obey their bodies.

MY TOP FIVE WORLD'S FITTEST YOU CARDIO ACTIVITIES

1. _____
2. _____
3. _____
4. _____
5. _____

Activities for All Seasons

There's a season for all of your outdoor activities. Some of these activities can be done all year round, depending on your specific climate. I've listed them here according to my own personal preferences. For instance, I really enjoy hiking in the fall when the leaves are changing color and there's a little chill in the air. But hiking is one of those activities you can do all year long.

Spring	Summer	Fall	Winter
In-line skating	Swimming	Running	Cross-country skiing
Tennis	Kayaking	Hiking	Downhill skiing
Walking	Volleyball		Snowboarding
	Cycling		

2. Strength Training

The second component of my "Shock Your Body" program is strength training. With these activities you'll be learning how to shock your muscles in ways that cardio activities can't do as effectively. While cardio activities build endurance, strength training builds up your muscles. What's great about muscle is that it fires up your metabolism. The more lean muscle tissue you have, the greater your metabolic rate and therefore the more calories you'll burn. Losing weight isn't enough; you have to replace that lost weight with muscle. Research shows that if you lose weight from just changing your eating habits without doing any physical activity, nearly a third of that weight will be from muscle rather than fat. It's the muscle weight you want to keep and fat you want to lose. The reason is that muscle is living, active tissue that eats up calories. Fat is inactive and takes up space. That's why you would rather have muscle than fat. It's important to build your muscles at the same time you are losing weight. With my core strength-training activities you'll see described in Appendix B, you'll get these benefits:

1. Improve your bones and joints
2. Help prevent injury such as bone-breaking falls
3. Build a toned, tighter physique
4. Avoid muscle loss, especially if your goal is to lose weight
5. Reduce your body fat
6. Reduce your blood cholesterol and blood fats
7. Improve your posture

These are some special tips for women:

- Do some whole-body lifts such as squats, lunges, standing press, or dead lifts, because these stress the long bones and help prevent osteoporosis.
- Avoid lifting heavy weights during pregnancy, because the hormone relaxin softens tendons and ligaments.
- Women generally have stronger abdominal muscles but are weaker than men in the upper-body area. Women should concentrate on upper-body strength.

Strength and the FIT Equation

So how do you keep lifting weights interesting and fun? That's the question I always get from my clients. Up and down, back and forth—there's nothing terribly exciting about lifting weights. That's why you have to constantly change up your routine and switch things around. But how do you do that? Simple. The FIT Equation lets you vary things in your weight routine so that you don't get bored. And not only that, it will help you "Shock Your Body" to reach new levels of fitness.

The first variable you'll be changing around is the Frequency. The Frequency combines two important strength-training concepts. A Repetition or "Rep" is the number of times you complete one motion of an activity. A "Set" is the number of times you complete consecutive motions of that same activity. So for example, when I say "ten reps and three sets" of Push-ups, this is what it means. You'll do ten push-ups, that's one set. Do another ten push-ups, that's two sets. Do ten more and that's three sets. As you advance, the Frequency—Reps and Sets—will change around quite a bit.

You'll also be varying the Intensity. This is a little harder to explain because it's so subjective. You see, Intensity is a feeling more than a prescribed quantitative number, like reps or sets. If you've never lifted weights before, at first it might be hard to gauge your intensity. But even if you have, I want you to think about your intensity in a completely different way. I don't want you to just go through the motions of lifting the weight, but really focus on the effort you're using. My intensity scale will help guide you:

WORLD'S FITTEST MAN STRENGTH INTENSITY SCALE

1. no activity
2. an easy lift with no muscle fatigue
3. a little muscle fatigue on the last few reps
4. a lot of muscle fatigue on the last few reps
5. complete muscle fatigue—your muscles are burning up on the last rep

The other variable you'll be aware of is Time, which is the amount of time you'll be resting after each set of an activity. The less time you have to rest, the harder you'll be working. The more time you rest, the easier you'll be working out. To put it simply, short rest periods help build muscular endurance while longer rest periods are used to increase strength and power.

You'll also be varying the amount of weight that you use. But this will be different for everyone on the program. That's why you'll see a blank box when you start. When you begin, I want you to find a weight that's comfortable so that you can perform all of the exercises (reps and sets) without straining yourself. As you progress through the program you'll be gradually increasing the amount of weight so that you're constantly challenging yourself and pushing your limits.

Let's take a look at one of my own strength-training workouts to help you understand how the FIT Equation works in practice.

Activity	Frequency		Intensity	Time	weight
	Reps	Sets			
Dumbbell Bench Press	10	3	3	2	100 pounds
Dumbbell Flye	10	3	3	2	70 pounds

I begin my workout with the chest muscle group. The first strength-training activity is the Dumbbell Press. The FIT Equation tells me exactly how I'm going to do it. The Frequency is ten Reps and three Sets. The Intensity is 3 and Time is two minutes. So here's how I do it. I start my first ten Reps of the bench press going at it with a medium intensity level of 3. That means my muscles feel a little fatigued on the last few reps, seven through ten. After I finish the ten Reps, that's one set. Then, I take a little breather for two minutes. That's the Time variable. I look down at my watch and time it exactly. When the two minutes are up, I do my next Set of presses, then rest again for two minutes. After three sets I move on to the next activity, Dumbbell Flye.

The 10 Percent Rule

Generally, you'll be increasing the weight about 5–10 percent when you can perform a set of the exercise for one or two above the number of reps. So, if you're doing a Dumbbell Bench Press set of ten reps with twenty-pound dumbbells and can successfully complete eleven or twelve reps without feeling any strain, you're ready to increase the weight. The next time try a twenty-five-pound dumbbell. You'll obviously be constrained by the weights available at your gym or at home. But I'd rather you work with a lighter weight than a heavier one. If it's too heavy, you may be sacrificing proper form and therefore risking injury.

The Perfect Rep

It's important that you focus on each and every repetition of each and every strength-training activity. To do this you should make each rep what I call "the Perfect Rep." This is a technique that I use in my own training and really helps me to get the maximum benefit from my workout. All you have to remember is "up two . . . down four." It works like this: When you lift the weight and go against gravity, count slowly to two (one thousand one . . . one thousand two works fine). When you lower the weight and have gravity on your side, count slowly down from four (four, three, two, one).

You'll see I've included this technique in just about all of my core strength-training activities (see Appendix B). As an example, let's take a closer look at the Dumbbell Bench Press on page 211. Here's how I do it. First, I will lift the weight slowly for two counts. When I reach the top of the movement, I pause and lower slowly for four counts. "Up for two . . . down for four." Say that to yourself a few times—all you have to do is count. I know it will take some practice to completely get the hang of "the Perfect Rep." For me, slow and steady really does win the race. Most of my clients are used to racing through their strength-training activities without even thinking. When I explain "the Perfect Rep" technique, they balk at how hard it is. Once they get used to the technique, they tell me they can really feel and see a difference. It's the best way to get the most results from your time spent doing weights.

Breathe!

It's okay to hold your breath when you're swimming underwater, but it's not a good thing when you're lifting weights. Throughout the movements that I show you, you'll want to maintain a steady breathing rhythm. I can't tell you how many clients come to me not knowing this. For years they've been holding their breath. In extreme cases this could cause a heart attack or a stroke, because there's simply not enough blood flowing to and from your heart. It puts excessive pressure on your chest and abdomen. More generally, if you hold your breath, you'll just feel dizzy and faint. Of course, that might just give you another excuse to stop. Here's the technique I'd like you to use: Exhale when you're lifting the weights and going against gravity (when you're doing the "up-for-two" movement). Inhale when you're returning the weights to the starting position (when you're doing the "down-for-four" movement).

Why Push/Pull?

The basis of my program is a set of core strength activities that work every major muscle group in your body. But you won't be working the same muscles every day and never more than three days per week. Not only do you need to let your muscles rest between workouts, but you don't want to spend hours and hours just lifting weights. To be honest, who has the time for that? The way I divide up the strength-training activities is called "Push/Pull." The Push muscles consist of your chest, shoulders, and triceps. The Pull muscles are your back and biceps. The reason why I divide it up this way is because all the muscles in the Push and Pull group are synergistic—that is, they work together. For instance, you can't work the chest muscles without also working your shoulders and triceps. You can't work your back muscles without also working your biceps. When you work them together like this, you really get the most out of your workout.

The Home/Gym Version

If you decide to do my program at home, then you'll need some basic equipment, which I describe for you on page 44. Most of the strength-training activities are the same whether you do them at home or at the gym (provided you have the proper home equipment). These have the designation "Home/Gym Version." Some activities, however, use equipment that you'll be more likely to find at the gym, like a cable leg press or lat pulldown machine. If you're working out at home, don't despair, I've provided an alternative "Home Version" of these activities. They work basically the same muscles as the "Gym Version," but use your home equipment instead of those big machines you find at the gym.

Now, this is really important. Just because I've designated an activity as a "Home Version" doesn't mean you can't do it at the gym. If you are doing my program at the gym, I really encourage you to try out some of the "Home Version" activities. By doing these versions you'll add more variation to your workout. And as I keep saying, variation is the key to continually "Shock Your Body." If you are working out at home, you might want to get a day pass to your local gyms (most gyms let you work out for a day, without getting a yearly membership, for a very nominal fee). Or, you might see if a friend who has a gym membership can take you along for the day as a guest. Either way, a day at the gym using the special equipment there can add variety and spice up your workout. While you're at the gym you might even want to try a special class like spinning or yoga.

3. Stretching

More than anything, flexibility and stretching get overlooked. I hear it all the time from my clients: "Joe, really, do I have to stretch? I'm not really burning off calories, so what does it matter?" I tell them it's crucial to stretch. With all of the strength and cardio activities you'll be doing during the program, your muscles will shorten and stiffen. That's completely normal. What stretching does is protect your muscles and even joints from injury during all this activity. But don't just take my word for it. The ACSM thinks so too. Stretching is part of their general exercise recommendations, advising it be performed for all the major muscle groups at least two to three times per week. In my program you'll be stretching six days a week. That's how strongly I feel about the importance of stretching. It really doesn't take that much time and helps you feel great all day long. Besides preventing injury, stretching has all of these benefits:

1. Improves your blood circulation
2. Improves air exchange in your lungs, or your ability to take in oxygen
3. Helps prevent back pain
4. Decreases muscle soreness after exercise and recover faster
5. Improves your physical performance in activities
6. Keeps your muscles feeling younger

Before or After?

There's been much debate about the best time to stretch. I'm sure we can all remember our high school gym teacher instructing us to touch our toes at the beginning of gym class. Research shows that stretching before your workout doesn't do much good, and actually can do some harm. When you try to stretch muscles that are cold and tight, you run the risk of injury. I recommend stretching at the end of your workout, after you complete your cardio or strength-training activities. That is when your muscles are warm and supple, a perfect time to stretch them.

Holding It

There are many different types of stretching techniques. The one that I find the most beneficial and least likely to cause straining is a simple "static" stretch. In a "static" stretch you simply hold the movement. That means no bouncing or moving once you get into the stretch. By holding a stretch, you increase the length of the muscle, helping to prevent injury and soreness. You should feel tension, not pain, when you stretch. Pain indicates that you're straining the muscle and that's not good for your body.

I recommend holding each stretch for a minimum of fifteen seconds. That's really the bare minimum, any less time and you won't get any real benefits. When I stretch, I usually hold for about thirty seconds, sometimes longer. I know that sounds like a long time, but after putting all that stress on your muscles by either strength training or cardio, you need time to lengthen and stretch them. I also recommend that you repeat each stretch twice, although doing it once is better than nothing. The second time you stretch the muscle, you can actually go deeper and get a more intense stretch.

The World's Fittest Man's Total Body Stretch

My stretching routine consists of thirteen simple movements you'll see listed in Appendix C. I can't stress enough the importance of stretching. As you've read from my story, I do a lot of intense and sometimes crazy things to my body. I'll be the first to admit that running 135 miles through the desert is not for the faint of heart. It can definitely take its toll. Without stretching my body completely after each and every workout, I wouldn't be where I am today. I honestly believe that.

That's why my "Shock Your Body" program includes a total body stretch every day you work out. You will perform those twelve stretches after each and every workout, no matter what. I call it "the World's Fittest Man's Total Body Stretch." If you're short on time, I'd rather you skip one of the strength-training activities or cut five or ten minutes off your cardio workout to complete the stretching routine. Better to be safe and free from injury than sorry later. It's no fun sitting on the sidelines.

Relax Your Mind

Your stretching workout is a time not only to release tension in your muscles, but also to release tension in your mind. It's a time to let go of the stresses of the day and just relax into the stretch. I like to think of stretching as almost a meditation in motion. When I'm training really hard, like a long run or bike ride, I'm totally focused on the activity itself and the intensity of it all. Stretching afterward calms me down and releases all that adrenaline and tension.

So much of stretching is about breathing. When I'm working with clients to show them a stretch, I always ask them, "Are you breathing?" More often than not they're holding their breath. When you do a stretch, make sure to breathe out when going into the stretch and inhale when coming out of the stretch. While you're holding the stretch, take a full inhalation—filling up your lungs completely with each breath. This simple breathing technique also lets you go farther into the movement.

Throw in the Towel

You can also add variety to your stretches by adding a towel to your stretching routine. With a towel you might be able to get a deeper or more intense stretch than just with your hands. I'm pretty flexible—

but generally men aren't as flexible as women to begin with. I'll use a towel to pull myself forward. Take a look at the Seated Toe Touch on page 246. I find it difficult sometimes to actually touch my toes. What I'll do is hook a towel around my foot so that I can pull forward and feel the hamstring stretch a little bit deeper.

Where Should I "Shock My Body"?

My "Shock Your Body" program can be done in a gym or at home—you choose. Many of my clients prefer to work out at home because it's more convenient, efficient, and private. It's right there in your house, so you have no excuse. If you decide to choose the home option, you're going to need what's listed below, at the bare minimum. The cardio activities are a vital part of my program, so make sure you're able to do a few of the outdoor activities all year round. If not, you'll need to invest some money in home cardio equipment like a simple treadmill or elliptical trainer. These are the ultimate basics for setting up a home gym:

- *Chin-up Bar.* You can get a great chin-up bar for around $15. These are easy to install in just about any doorway. You can leave the bar or just put it up for your workouts. Better yet, you can even take it with you to the office or when you travel.
- *Jump Rope.* It's amazing how such a simple and inexpensive piece of equipment can give you one of the world's best cardio workouts. A basic jump rope costs about $5. More expensive ones cost up to $20. For that price you get leather handles for a better grip and ball bearings for a smoother workout.
- *Multipurpose Bench.* This will probably be the biggest piece of equipment you'll need for getting your home gym off the ground. There are many different types of benches, but I recommend a bench that gives you three positions: flat, incline, and decline. You can get one of these for under $100. The incline and decline features cost a little bit more, but you'll really get your money's worth

over time. A basic flat bench will cost you less, but you'll probably outgrow it very quickly.

- *Dumbbells.* A good set of dumbbells will be the mainstay of your home gym. There's no getting around this piece of equipment. There are two different types of dumbbells. One type is a fixed-weight dumbbell such as five pounds. If you're going to choose this option, you're going to need at least six different weights. The other kind is called adjustable-weight dumbbells. I recommend this option because it's less expensive and more versatile. You can buy a forty-pound set for around $50. The set usually includes two bars with collars, four five-pound weights, and four two-and-a-half-pound weights. Perfect for both men and women, beginners and advanced. As you get stronger, you can even purchase additional weights to add to your set.
- *Exercise Mat.* To keep yourself off the floor you might want to invest in an exercise mat. This is an optional piece of equipment, but it's probably money well spent. You can get a basic mat for around $15. If you want a thicker mat with lots of cushioning, you'll spend a little more.

There's No Excuse

If you decide to choose the gym option, I strongly suggest that you have a "fitness backup plan" in case you can't make it to the gym that day. For the backup plan you'll need a jump rope or pair of running shoes to do some high-intensity cardio. For weights you can use whatever is around the house or in the garage. I call them "household dumbbells" (see chart on page 46). For a bench you can use a piano bench or place a sturdy board between two chairs. Here are a few of my favorite "household dumbbells." I'm sure you can find your own, just make sure whatever object you choose has a strong, comfortable grip.

JOE'S HOUSEHOLD DUMBBELLS

Product	Weight
50 oz. of liquid laundry detergent	4 pounds
½ gallon of milk	5 pounds
60 oz. of liquid laundry detergent	6 pounds
100 oz. of liquid laundry detergent	7 pounds
1 gallon of water	9 pounds
1 gallon of liquid laundry detergent	10 pounds

"Outside the Box" Workouts

On Saturday, the sixth day of each week of the program, I've designed some special workouts to give your body a chance to think "outside the box." By that I mean fitness activities to get you away from your normal routine, whether you work out at the gym or at home. These are unique workouts you do right in your own backyard with little or no equipment. It's also a chance for you to escape from your usual location and get a real change of scenery, like a playground or baseball field. What's more, these workouts will "Shock Your Body" in a totally different way through what's called a "total body circuit"—a fat-burning combination of both strength and cardio training.

A total body circuit is a series of activities you do one right after the other with little or no break in between. Some of the activities will be from my core strength-training movements. The difference here is that you do them with much lighter weights and higher reps. Performing these activities with low weight and high reps helps your body build muscle endurance rather than muscle mass. Mixed in with the strength training, you'll do a series of cardio activities like running, walking, jumping, climbing stairs, even skipping. All of these can get your heart beating faster. Finally, some of the activities may seem new but they're actually based on simple and familiar calisthenic movements.

Here's how it all works. Like all my other workouts, you'll start off with a five-minute warm-up to get your heart rate up. Then, I'll give you a list of eight to ten activities that you'll do one right after the other, and that's called your circuit. With some of the activities I'll really want you to "Shock Your Body" with a technique called "till muscle fatigue." What that means is instead of doing predetermined reps and sets like you do on the other days of my program, you'll perform the activity until your muscles can't take it anymore—"till muscle fatigue." As you see, in these workouts I'm trying to get you out of your regular "comfort zones" and push you to new fitness levels.

After you complete the circuit of activities, you'll rest for several minutes, then do the circuit again, depending on how you feel. If you're at a higher fitness level, you can probably do four or five sets of the circuit. If you're just starting out, then one or two might be more appropriate for your level of fitness. You can—and should—listen to your body and adjust the workouts to your own needs.

For instance, in the first week of the program I've designed one of these circuits to do on a playground. I call it the "Power Playground Workout" (see page 106). This one is very popular with my clients. When I tell them we're going to a playground for a workout they can't believe it. "A playground is just for kids," Judy, one of my clients, told me. She just couldn't believe that you didn't have to go to the gym to get fit. Once she started the playground workout, she said it made her feel like a little kid again. "This feels more like playing than working out," she told me. After forty-five minutes I had to pull her off the monkey bars because our session was over. She didn't even realize how fast the time had gone—and didn't want to stop. Just a note about weather. If the weather makes it impossible for you to go outside, then try to find a suitable indoor location, like a school gym or indoor track. If that doesn't work, and you're really stuck, substitute a thirty- to forty-five-minute cardio workout. Doing something is always better than doing nothing. My classes meet outside year round, rain, snow, or shine. Many of my clients love jogging in the rain or playing in the snow. Remember to have *fun* on these days.

Putting It All Together

Now that you've seen what the activities are and how to do them using the FIT Equation, you're ready to put it all together. You'll see that it's all easy and simple to follow. I've designed a workout for you each day of my four-week "Shock Your Body" program. The workouts for these four weeks will all last about forty-five minutes, so there's really no excuse not to do them. Some days will even be a little less. I've also separated the cardio activities from the strength ones. You won't be doing cardio and strength on the same day; that way your muscles have adequate time to rest between workouts. You will be stretching with my World's Fittest Man's Total Body Stretch every day you work out. Sunday will be your rest day, with no workout at all.

If you miss a day, don't make a big deal about it. And don't try to make up for it the next day by doing a double workout. Simply pick up the next day where you left off. I know we all have busy schedules with jobs and families. Interruptions are bound to come up. But it's important that you follow the program as closely as possible, at least in the beginning. It will take you some time to get used to following the FIT Equation.

THE POWER OF POSITIVE EATING

CHAPTER 4

DO'S AND DON'TS

Remember, my program is about simple, small changes. I don't believe in diets because they simply don't work. They didn't work for me, and, yes, I've tried them all, and most of the experts agree that they won't work for you either. What works for me is focusing on eating, not dieting. Diets make you think in the negative: I can't eat this, I can't eat that. That's why my plan is about everyday eating strategies, ones that I used to become the World's Fittest Man and ones you can use too. I do not take a lot of special supplements, or drink expensive muscle protein shakes. I eat normal, everyday food you can find in your average grocery store. For me it's all about do's, not don'ts. Eating is about the do's and dieting is about the don'ts.

My eating program is simple. It's ten simple do's that are easy to follow. I call it the "Power of Positive Eating" because eating has to be a positive experience, otherwise you'll fall back into those bad habits that you're trying to change. I believe that you're not going to change eating habits overnight. When I was losing weight it took me a while to learn how to eat healthily. And that's the key. You want to change your lifestyle so you can lose weight and keep it off. Those fad diets and gimmicks may help you in the short term, but you'll never keep off that weight. I still fall off the healthy-eating wagon every once in a while and have to reevaluate myself. That's why I've designed my "Power of Positive Eating" program. It's a ten-step plan for changing what you eat and how you eat it. What makes my eating program different is that it's about small victories and gradual changes. I've found that most people I've trained who want to lose weight try to make radical changes immediately. While I admire their enthusiasm, changing everything at once just doesn't work. Change must happen slowly, over time.

You'll see I have a list of ten "Eating Do's." Now, please don't look at the list and say to yourself, *That's too many things.* You're right, for one day it's way too much to follow. But gradually, over the course of my four-week program, you'll be incorporating all of these small changes into your lifestyle.

CALORIES COUNT

We're fat because we eat too much. That's all there is to it. Some people blame it on eating too many carbohydrates. Others blame it on low-fat food. And some blame a problem with their thyroids. Of course, those things are part of the problem. But let's get real for a minute. Calories count, and according to United States Department of Agriculture (USDA) data, since 1984 the daily calorie intake for each person is up 500. What that means is that over the course of a year, if you're not doing any physical activity, you're adding inches to your belly. So where are those 500 calories coming from? It's hard to be exactly sure, but USDA figures show that during this same time period, there's been a 39 percent increase in calories from refined grains like white flour and white rice, a 32 percent increase from added fats, and a 24 percent increase from sugar. And most of that sugar is coming from soft drinks.

So you'll see in my "Power of Positive Eating" program that I address all of those problems: refined grains, added fats, and white sugar.

I'll show you how to substitute fiber-filling whole grains for nutrient-lacking white grains through a simple "Grain Exchange" formula. And I'll show you how to gradually reduce dietary saturated fat. I call it "Less Fat, Lose Fat."

WHY DIETING DOESN'T WORK

At one time or another most people have tried a "diet" to lose weight. Yes, even I've tried them all. If you're like me, then you've probably met with little success, much disappointment, and ultimately frustration. The term *diet* actually refers to what we eat, not a process of weight loss. Restricting the type and quantity of food we eat for periods of time and then returning to our normal eating habits doesn't promote weight loss. This form of dieting may actually make future weight loss more difficult by changing the rate your body naturally burns calories and fat. Any modification or change to your eating habits needs to be a change to promote weight loss and provide real health benefits. Lifestyle changes are the only proven way to maintain and lose weight. Eating a balanced diet can provide the nutrients necessary to power your body. But eating too much will cause the body to store fat. Working out to help increase the calories your body burns will balance your food intake with the calories needed to provide energy for living. I know this sounds like common sense, but many people try to make this more complicated than it is.

DIETING CONTROVERSIES

One of the main reasons dieting doesn't work is that after you've restricted your eating for whatever period of time, you go back to your regular habits. One of the most popular diets out there today is the Atkins diet, which restricts the amount of carbohydrates you eat, but allows you to eat just about all the fats and protein you want. I'm sure you've heard stories about the amazing amount of weight people have lost on this diet. His book, *Dr. Atkins' New Diet Revolution,* has sold millions of copies, so you'd expect to hear about millions of people who've lost weight. Instead, it's just the opposite; the obesity epidemic has gotten worse and worse. I had a friend on the diet who ate burgers (no buns), and cheese and greasy bacon. He lost forty pounds but soon after gained back fifty.

What you maybe haven't heard is that some research shows these low-carbohydrate/high-protein diets, like the Atkins diet, are less successful over the long term and may even be hazardous to your health. What some researchers have found is that protein-rich foods high in fat increase the risk of heart disease and type 2 diabetes. Not only that, the diet severely strains the kidneys, increasing the risk of kidney stones while at the same time increasing the risk of bone loss.

Besides the Atkins diet there are lots of other diet fads out there. Sometimes quick-fix diets are hard to spot. It's easy to get taken in. Here are some easy ways the American Dietetic Association suggests to help you sort out fact from fad:

- Recommendations that promise a quick fix.
- Dire warnings of dangers from a single product or regimen.
- Claims that sound too good to be true.
- Recommendations based on a single study.
- Recommendations made to help sell a product.
- "You'll keep it off forever."
- "Weight loss is effortless."

And you won't have too much trouble finding false and misleading nutrition and dieting claims. A report from the FDA found that nearly half of all weight-loss advertising had at least one false or misleading claim. What's more, they found that this type of deceptive advertising has dramatically increased over the last decade.

Here are some weight-loss gimmicks and claims that you may have seen. They certainly get my attention, but unfortunately, they're not true:

- "Lose ten pounds in eight days."
- "Starts to work immediately."
- "No exercise and eat as much as you want. The more you eat, the more you lose."
- "You can eat as much as you want and still lose weight."

FATS

What Are Fats?

Let's start with fats. There's much talk about fats these days. Fat is a necessary and important part of your diet. What you need to know is that while some fats are actually good for you, the majority, the ones that you're probably used to eating, should be eliminated from your diet. These fats are called "saturated" fats and you'll find them in butter, heavy cream, lard, and foods of animal origin. Saturated fat doesn't just make you fat by adding lots of extra calories to your diet; there's also scientific evidence that this type of fat increases your chances of having a heart attack and getting high blood pressure.

The fats that are good for you are "unsaturated" fats like olive oil and peanut oil. They are mostly found in foods of plant origin and some seafood. These types of fats are also called "monounsaturated" and "polyunsaturated" fats. There's some great news about olive oil, one of the monounsaturated fats. Research shows that olive oil may actually help you lose body fat and improve your heart- and blood-vessel health. That's why you'll see that so many of the recipes here and meals in this book include olive oil. If you're cooking with olive oil and peanut oil already, that's great. In any case I'll also show you how to prepare some great-tasting meals by using some surprising low-fat, healthy alternatives to saturated fat.

Another type of unsaturated fat that's good for your health is the omega-3 fatty acid. These fats are found mostly in seafood, especially tuna and salmon, but also in some oils like soybean and canola, as well as green leafy vegetables and walnuts. Research shows that increasing the amount of omega-3 fatty acids can have a beneficial effect on the health of your heart by reducing the chances of getting a heart attack. Some other potential benefits include prevention of abnormal heart rhythms, decreased risk of clots, and lower triglyceride levels. You'll see that many of the meals in my plan include salmon, tuna, and other seafood. Studies show that eating just two servings of fish each week can lower your risk of coronary heart disease.

There's one fat that's the absolute worst, and you should avoid it at all costs. You won't see this fat at all in my program. It's called "trans fatty acid," or more commonly "trans fat." These fats are made artificially from partially hydrogenated vegetable oils, and they are almost twice as bad for you as saturated fats, which means they are twice as likely to cause heart disease, clog your arteries, and increase your chances of having a stroke.

The big problem is that manufacturers love to use trans fat because it's cheaper and easier. You'll find trans fats in many baked goods like cookies and cakes; it's what makes cookies have that buttery taste and gives icing its firmness. Restaurants, especially fast-food restaurants, use trans fat to fry foods and make them more crisp. Luckily, things are starting to change. The FDA is now requiring food labels to include trans fat amounts. I'll show you how to spot it later on in this chapter.

Of course, you're not going to be losing weight by cutting back on "bad" fat alone. You're going to have to cut back on your calorie intake and slowly increase the amount of physical exercise you do. But fat, whether good or bad, is the most concentrated source of calories in your diet. As I said before, fat has more than twice as many calories, gram for gram, as carbohydrates and protein.

Good Fats		Bad Fats	
Monounsaturated fats	Polyunsaturated fats	Saturated	Trans fat
olive oil, canola oil, peanut oil, cashews, almonds, peanut butter, avocado	vegetable oil, safflower oil, fish oil (this includes omega-3 fatty acids)	whole milk, cheese, ice cream, red meat, coconut oil	most margarines, vegetable shortening, partially hydrogenated vegetable oil, deep-fried chips, many fast foods

CARBS

Why Do We Need Carbs?

If you think of your body as an amazing piece of machinery, then you're going to need fuel to keep it running. Carbohydrates are the primary source of fuel for your body. Since you'll be increasing your activity level at least for the next four weeks on my program, carbohydrates are really going to give you the energy to keep moving. Carbohydrates also keep your blood sugar at the right levels and your brain functioning properly. When you're at work, you may feel that lull at around three in the afternoon. It probably means your blood sugar is a little low and you need a carbohydrate-rich snack to refuel your body for the next two or three hours of work. Snacks are an important part of my eating program. You're not going to want to skimp on these healthy treats.

What Are Good Carbs/Bad Carbs?

Let me start by saying that I love carbohydrates. And, yes, they are good for you. The misunderstanding about carbohydrates is that they are all lumped together. The fact is, not all carbohydrates are created equal and that's why I think it's important to spend a little time explaining the differences between what I call "good carbs/bad carbs."

The Importance of Whole Grains

While not all carbs are created equal, neither are all grains. White bread and white flour are made up of refined grains, that is, they've been processed to take out all the good, healthy nutrients. I try to avoid white bread products and white pasta as much as possible. Instead, I include whole grains or unrefined grains whenever I can. Most important, whole grains are an excellent source of fiber in your diet. As I said before, fiber gives you that "full" feeling so you end up eating less. Fiber has also been shown to have a great effect on your health. Whole-grain foods may lower the risk of heart disease, protect against type 2 diabetes, improve your gastrointestinal health, and reduce your risk to certain types of cancer. What's more, research shows that people who consume lots of whole-grain foods have a lower body mass index (BMI).

Grain Exchange

There are some easy ways to add whole grains to your diet. I call it "Grain Exchange." It's a simple way to substitute whole grains for white flour and highly refined grains. The way I do it is easy. One simple "Grain Exchange" I do is start off the day with a whole-grain or bran cereal instead of Fruit Loops or Sugar Frosted Flakes. An easy way to tell if it's whole grain is by taking a look at the fiber count. Check out the ingredients to know what you're putting in your body. If the serving has more than five grams of fiber, then you know you're eating a whole, unrefined grain. For bread I make sure I'm eating whole-wheat or multigrain bread. Now, be careful, some of the breads that you see in your local grocery store may say that they're whole wheat but are not much better for you than white bread. Here's a trick that I use to make sure the bread is really whole wheat. First, look at the ingredients list: If you see "whole-wheat flour," then you know you're on the right track. Then, take a look at the food label. If the fiber content is around five grams per slice, then go for it; you've got yourself a healthy, whole-grain bread. Believe it or not, pasta is another way you can add whole grains and fiber to your diet. If you're like me, you probably grew up on huge bowls of spaghetti and macaroni. Unfortunately, that pasta wasn't whole grain, so I'm sure it had something to do with my gaining some weight. Here's a great trick: Simply substitute whole-wheat pasta for the white-flour kind. It's now so popular that you can find it in your regular grocery store right next to the white flour pasta.

OTHER SIMPLE WHOLE-GRAIN SUBSTITUTIONS:

Instead of that:	Try this:
Sweetened corn flakes cereal	Raisin Bran, Mini-Wheats, Oatmeal
Bagel or white bread	Seven-grain or multigrain bread
Flour tortilla	Whole-wheat tortilla
White rice	Brown rice
Regular pasta	Whole-wheat, buckwheat, or spinach pasta
White pita	Whole-wheat pita
Ritz or saltine crackers	Nabisco Triscuits, whole-wheat crackers
Chocolate-chip cookie	Whole-wheat fig cookie

Glycemic Index and Carbs

So how do you determine which "carbs" are good and which are bad? Simply put, nutritionists have come up with an index of foods and how those foods affect the level of sugar in your blood. It's called the "glycemic index." In scientific terms it measures how much carbohydrate contained in the food raises the level of blood glucose and need for insulin over two hours. To you and me it measures how fast that carbohydrate, whether it's a bagel or banana, gets digested. You know that sugar rush you get right after you eat a candy bar? Well, after that candy bar is digested, all the sugar goes straight into your bloodstream. The candy bar fills you up for a little bit, but when that sugar rush is over, you'll probably feel even hungrier. I know it's crude, but that candy bar acts somewhat like an addictive drug. People who do drugs feel great for a few minutes and then crash. Once they come down they instantly crave more. That candy bar works in some of the same ways. A candy bar, or anything that's processed with lots of refined sugar, has a high glycemic index. These are the foods you're going to want to stay away from, since they add lots of calories but don't really fill you up. On my eating program I'll show you how to load up your diet with healthy carbs with a low glycemic index. That is, foods that will keep your blood sugar more controlled. For example, rather than a candy bar for a snack you'll do better with a banana or another piece of fruit. It's not just a caloric difference; the banana has a lower glycemic index. So after your body digests that piece of fruit, your blood sugar will not shoot up and you will feel more satisfied.

Why is all this glycemic index stuff important to you? How will it help you become "the World's Fittest You"? Without getting too technical, research shows that a sharp rise in blood sugar, caused by eating high-glycemic-index foods, actually can make you fat. Here's what happens. The rise in blood sugar causes a surge of insulin. That in turn promotes your dietary fat to turn into fat cells. Those fat cells eventually become the bulges that you might see on your hips, thighs, and midsection. More than changing the way your body looks, high-glycemic-index foods increase your risk for type 2 diabetes and cardiac disease. Low-glycemic-index foods, the ones you should eat, help to lower your triglycerides and LDL (bad cholesterol), as well as promote a healthier ratio of total cholesterol to HDL.

Glycemic Index of Some Common Foods

Food	GI Value
Yogurt, low-fat	20
Peanuts	21
Red kidney beans	27
Cherries	32
Grapefruit	36
Lentils	41
Skim milk	46
Pear	53
Tomato soup	54
Bran cereal	60
Peach	60
Orange	63
Grapes	66
Mixed-grain bread	69
Jam	70
Ice cream, low-fat	71
Orange juice	74
Banana	77
Sweet potato	77
Sweet corn	78
Brown rice	79
Oatmeal cookies	79
White rice	83
Split pea soup	86
Ice cream	87

Food	GI Value
Raisins	91
Pineapple	94
Croissant	96
Wheat crackers	96
White bagel	103
Corn chips	105
French fries	107
Donut	108
White bread	112
Jelly beans	114
Pretzels	116
Potato	117
Cornflakes	119

PROTEIN

Good Sources of Protein

You're going to need protein because it provides the primary ingredient for your body to build and repair muscle, blood, skin, and other tissue. The best sources of protein are ones that are lean and low in saturated fat. You also want proteins that are going to give you all the amino acids you need to build muscle. I usually stick to the basics like chicken, fish (tuna and salmon), and turkey. If you're going to have beef, that's okay, too, but make sure it's a lean cut such as the eye of round, top round, and round tip. Surprisingly, these cuts have about 150 calories per three-ounce serving, and less than five grams of saturated fat.

Dairy products are great sources of protein too. But like beef you're going to want to choose ones that are low in saturated fat. For milk, use skim or low fat. For eggs, I usually separate out the whites from the yolk. I know it's a little messy, but you're going to get a very lean source of protein without all the saturated fat. At first you might want to try this variation: combine three egg whites with one yolk for your omelet. That one yolk adds a little more flavor. Cheese is also a good source of protein. But be careful. First, choose a fat-free or low-fat variety. Most cheeses like American, cheddar, and Swiss have a low-fat or fat-free version. But also pay attention to the portion. If you buy cheese in a block, keep track of your portions. It's easy to go overboard when you cut the cheese yourself. Instead, I suggest buying individually wrapped cheese. That way it's easier to tell the portion size than by cutting it yourself. And don't forget yogurt. There are lots of great-tasting low- and fat-free brands. Most people think that yogurt is only for breakfast. I love to eat it as a snack during the day and even blend it with some fresh berries and ice for a delicious frozen parfait as dessert.

There are other sources of protein that you'll see in the meal plans here. One of my favorites is black beans (you'll see it's on my list of World's Fittest Foods). Beans, unlike meat and cheese, are incomplete proteins. Peanut butter and tofu are some other examples. That doesn't mean you should avoid them. It does mean that you'll have to combine them with another food to get the complete amino acids.

Dangers of Eating Too Much Protein

Getting enough protein is important, but eating too much can be dangerous. It can lead to serious digestive problems and a condition called "ketosis." Too much protein, especially for women, can have a harmful effect on your bones too. One study found that women who ate more than ninety-five grams of protein each day had more broken wrists than those eating the average amount.

FOOD MYTHS VERSUS FITTEST MAN'S FOOD FACTS

Now that you know the facts, what about all those myths about food? You wouldn't believe how much time I spend with my clients trying to dispel myths about dieting and weight loss. There's so much bad information floating around that it's hard to figure out what's fact and what's fiction. These are some of the common myths about food and dieting I see and hear most frequently:

Food Myth

Eating more protein will help you build muscle faster.

Fittest Man's Food Fact

If you're a bodybuilder who's training for a competition, then perhaps you should be concerned about the amount of protein you're eating. You're probably not one. By following my "Power of Positive Eating" program you'll build muscle, not by eating lots of extra protein, but by eating a balanced diet low in processed foods and high in fruits, vegetables, whole grains, and lean meats. At the same time you'll "Shock Your Body" with my total fitness program. As you increase the amount of physical activity, you'll want to make sure you are getting enough protein to maintain your muscles. Sorry to say, simply adding more protein to your diet won't give you bigger and stronger muscles. Again, this comes from a combination of hard work and proper eating habits.

Food Myth

"Health foods" are always good for you.

Fittest Man's Food Fact

This was one of the biggest surprises to me when I first started to lose weight and monitor what kinds of foods I was eating. I'd walk into a local health-food store or the "health-food" section of my local supermarket and think it was all good for me. In fact, unless you want organic food, you can find just about all the food that I recommend in my program in your local supermarket. These are some examples that many of my clients believed to be healthy but that, when you look at the nutritional content, really aren't:

Vegetable Chips or Crisps: If you think you're getting vegetables by eating a bag of these treats, think again. The bag shows tomatoes, squash, and other fresh vegetables, but the amount is so small they're used more for color than for nutritional value. With only slightly fewer calories than potato chips, you're better off with a fresh carrot or celery stick.

Bottled Health Juices: The health-food store is filled with a dizzying assortment of exotic juices. Apple strawberry. Cranberry mango. Kiwi passion fruit. They all sound very tasty and healthy. Right? Wrong. Even if the bottle says "100 percent juice," it's still loaded with lots of empty sugar calories. Unlike whole fruit, concentrated juices lack fiber, which fills you up and helps your digestion.

Yogurt-Covered: Yogurt is great for you when it's low-fat and served by itself. When raisins, peanuts, or pretzels are covered with yogurt, watch out. You're getting much more than you bargained for. Just check out the calories and fat in one cup of these:

- yogurt-covered peanuts: 921 calories, 73 g fat.
- yogurt-covered raisins: 750 calories, 14 g fat.
- yogurt-covered pretzels: 392 calories, 14 g fat.

Banana Chips: Don't be fooled by the word *banana.* They're more like chips than fruit. Just three ounces of these chips contain 450 calories, and are deep fried in coconut oil so they contain twenty-four grams of saturated fat—as many calories as two slices of Domino's deep-dish pizza or a large order of McDonald's french fries. My advice: If you're craving something banana flavored, stick to the real thing. It's only one hundred calories and will satisfy you more than a handful of banana chips.

Food Myth

Snacks before bedtime get converted directly to fat.

Fittest Man's Food Fact

I hear this one all the time. There's this big misconception about how eating snacks before going to bed will make you fat. That's not entirely true. Whether you eat a snack in the morning or right before hitting the pillow, your body will store extra calories as fat. It's not the time of day you eat the snack but how many calories are in the snack. Calories count no matter what time of day. This doesn't mean to wait until bedtime to throw down a bag of chocolate-chip cookies either.

Food Myth

The more carbohydrates you eat, the fatter you'll become.

Fittest Man's Food Fact

There's a widespread belief these days that carbohydrates make you fat. To be honest, many of my clients are now afraid to eat carbohydrates at all. They fear that by eating a piece of fruit or bowl of cereal, they will send those carbohydrates directly to their hips. "Joe, it's the carbs. All those carbs are making me fat," one of my clients kept telling me. Despite everyone's fears about carbohydrates making you fat, just the opposite is true. In fact, a USDA study of ten thousand adults showed that high-carbohydrate diets rich in whole-grain foods actually promote weight loss. Researchers split participants into four groups. One group got 30 percent of their calories from carbohydrates, the second 30–45 percent, the third 45–55 percent, and the fourth more than 55 percent. Surprisingly, the researchers found that the fourth group, the one with the highest percent of calories from carbohydrates, consumed three hundred fewer calories. Not only that, they got the most nutrients and achieved the lowest average body mass index. Like the research shows, I'm a case in point. I get most of my daily calories from complex carbohydrates, primarily whole grains, fruits, and vegetables.

Food Myth

A quick and easy way to knock off a few pounds is to skip meals.

Fittest Man's Food Fact

This is one of the oldest tricks in the book for those trying to lose weight. I've tried it myself too. Skip a meal and you save yourself a few hundred calories. It makes sense, in theory. Unfortunately, skipping meals actually works opposite to the way you'd expect. When you skip a meal, it makes you more hungry so you tend to overeat at the next meal. And it actually slows down your metabolic rate. Research shows that people who skip breakfast tend to be heavier than those who eat a nutritious breakfast. What's more, people who eat a balanced high-fiber breakfast eat less food later in the day.

Food Myth

Chewing on celery and carrots can burn off calories.

Fittest Man's Food Fact

To be honest, I'm not sure where this one comes from, but you can't burn off calories from chewing on celery and carrots. You might think you're doing a lot of activity moving your jaw up and down, but it's not enough to get your heart pumping and calories burning. Celery and carrots are healthy, low-calorie snacks, but don't eat an entire bag of baby carrots, for instance. That's two hundred calories. Portions still count, even if the food is healthy. And be very careful if carrots and celery are served next to sour cream or other kinds of high-fat dip. Each carrot covered with dip could have as many as three hundred calories.

Food Myth

You can't get fat by eating low-fat or nonfat foods.

Fat-Free/Reduced Fat	Calories	Regular	Calories
Reduced-fat peanut butter, 2 tbsp.	187	Regular peanut butter, 2 tbsp.	191
Reduced-fat chocolate-chip cookies, 3 cookies	118	Regular chocolate-chip cookies, 3 cookies	142
Fat-free fig cookies, 2 cookies	102	Regular fig cookies, 2 cookies	111
Nonfat vanilla frozen yogurt, ½ cup	100	Regular whole-milk vanilla frozen yogurt, ½ cup	104
Light vanilla ice cream, ½ cup	111	Regular vanilla ice cream, ½ cup	133
Low-fat granola cereal, ½ cup	213	Regular granola cereal, ½ cup	257
Baked tortilla chips, 1 oz.	113	Regular tortilla chips, 1 oz.	143
Low-fat cereal bar, 1 bar	130	Regular cereal bar, 1 bar	140

Fittest Man's Food Fact

Here's one that always gets me: "There's no fat in those cookies, so I can eat as many as I want." *Wrong!* Unfortunately, so many people have been misled by the myth of low-fat. Yes, saturated fat is bad for you, but *low-fat* or *fat-free* doesn't mean "calorie-free." In fact, many low-fat and fat-free foods have just as many calories as their fat-containing equivalents. Later on when you're following the meal plans, you'll see some low-fat items like low-fat yogurt and low-fat cheese. But that's not just because of the calories. It's because these low-fat items generally have less saturated fat. In some cases like salad dressing and mayonnaise, *low-fat* and *fat-free* do make a big difference, in terms of calories. Two tablespoons of some regular salad dressings have as many as two hundred calories, while the low-fat version of the same amount can have under fifty. If you're not sure, check the label. And check out the chart on page 66 comparing calorie content of some popular foods. Next time you reach for that fat-free cookie, take a quick look at the calorie count first.

"LESS FAT, LOSE FAT"

I'm sure you've tried many diets. Well, so have I. But with any diet the bottom line is that if you eat fewer calories than what your body needs, then you're going to lose weight. A lot of experts and dieticians try to make the equation harder than it actually is.

What I've discovered on my own and helping others get in shape is this: Dietary fat, whether it's saturated or unsaturated, is easy to limit from what you eat. By limiting fat, you're reducing the number of calories that enter your body. But don't just take my word for it. Research shows that people who lose weight and keep it off do so most successfully by eating fewer fatty foods.

Here's the reality. Fat has more calories per weight than any other type of food. It has nine calories per gram, while carbohydrates and proteins have four. By simply cutting back on fat you'll be able to eat

Instead of that:	Try this:
2 tbsp. butter	A bowl of high-fiber cereal with fresh strawberries
2 tbsp. lard	A cup of yogurt and a large banana
2 tbsp. cocoa butter	A cup of lentil soup, toast, and 20 carrot sticks
2 tbsp. margarine	A serving of my World's Fittest Man Dijon Mustard Chicken Nuggets (see recipe on page 267)
2 tbsp. corn oil	A serving of my World's Fittest Man Black Bean and Turkey Chili (see recipe on page 269)

more of other types of food that will really fill you up. So think of "Less Fat, Lose Fat" as getting more bang for your buck. In other words, you can eat more food that will really fill you up when you cut down on your calories from fat. What's more, dietary fat converts to body fat more efficiently than does protein or carbohydrates. So by making this small modification in your diet, eating *less fat,* you're really going to make it easier to *lose fat.*

Just to show you, the chart above tells you what you can eat in place of just two tablespoons of your favorite fat or fatty foods.

Let me be clear. You won't be cutting out all fats from your diet. Unsaturated fats like olive oil and omega-3 are an important part of the plan. Even with healthy fats, moderation is the key. Pouring two tablespoons of olive oil on your salad is still 240 calories no matter how you slice it. I just wanted to show you how easy it is to cut calories by making a few small changes in what you eat. Look how much food you can have instead of just two tablespoons of fat.

THE WORLD'S FITTEST YOU EATING GUIDE

Like me I'm sure you're familiar with the USDA food pyramid. You've probably seen it all over the place: from the backs of cereal boxes to bulletin boards in elementary-school classrooms. Since the 1980s, when the food pyramid first appeared, we have relied on these serving sizes and food selections to guide how much and what to eat. Now,

WORLD'S FITTEST YOU FOOD GUIDE

Food Type	Daily Portions	Examples of One Portion
"Good carbs"	6–9	A slice of multigrain bread, a small sweet potato, ½ cup brown rice, 1 cup bran flakes, 6 whole-wheat crackers, ½ cup black beans, 1 cup lentil soup
Meat and meat substitutes	2–4	A 4-oz. chicken breast, a 4-oz. salmon fillet, a 6-oz. can of water-packed tuna, 2 slices of cheese, ½ cup tofu
Fruit	3	1 apple, 1 cup strawberries, 1 banana, 1 cup blueberries
Vegetables	3–5	½ cup cooked broccoli, 1 cup mixed green salad, 1 cup cauliflower
Milk/dairy	2	1 cup skim milk, 8 oz. low-fat yogurt
"Good fat"	3–6 tsp.	1 tsp. olive oil, 1 tbsp. low-fat mayonnaise, 1 tbsp. low-fat salad dressing, 12 almonds, 1 tsp. peanut butter

it seems that the USDA food pyramid doesn't give you the complete picture.

What I've done, based on some of the latest diet and nutrition research, is clarify and update the USDA pyramid for my program so that it includes some important distinctions (see chart on page 69). Take fat, for instance. While the USDA pyramid advocates using fats "sparingly," not all fats are the same. When I say "Less Fat, Lose Fat," I'm really talking about cutting back on those harmful saturated fats from your diet.

You'll also see that I make a big distinction between carbohydrates. The USDA pyramid lumps them all together as the basis of the pyramid. In my program there are "good carbs" and "bad carbs." We'll build on this later, but for now you can see that you'll be eating six to nine portions of "good carbs" each day.

VITAMINS/SUPPLEMENTS

There's so much conflicting information about vitamins these days. One day it's this vitamin, the next day it's that one. And have you been to your local vitamin store lately? If you have, you've probably noticed the proliferation of supplements and vitamins making all sorts of claims—some that they promote "cardiovascular health," others that they "boost your metabolism," and others that they'll "block the fat." All this can be very confusing.

Does that mean you shouldn't be taking supplements at all? No. What I take, and many experts agree, is a basic multivitamin. Like the ones you find in your local pharmacy or supermarket. I used to believe, like many people, that you could get all your vitamins and minerals by just eating a healthy diet. But that thinking has changed, and now many doctors say that you should supplement your diet with a basic multivitamin.

Glucosamine and chondroitin are dietary supplements made from animal tissue. I take a recommended dosage that combines both chondroitin and glucosamine. (You should check the bottle for specific dosage recommendations.) While the FDA has not approved the safety or effectiveness of these supplements, I believe there is some compelling evidence that they can be good for you. Taken together, it's been widely reported that glucosamine and chondroitin can be effective in maintaining healthy joints and even preventing osteoarthritis. With all the running I do, there is an overall wear and tear on my bones and joints. I believe these supplements may help keep me in tip-top shape. Check with your doctor first, but I recommend it for you too.

THE POWER OF POSITIVE EATING: TEN STEPS TO HEALTHY EATING

Let's go back to that nutrition inventory you took in Chapter 2 and see how you did. Even if you did well, this part of my program is important to help you become "the World's Fittest You." These ten steps, what I call the "Power of Positive Eating," show you in simple terms how to eat healthy for the rest of your life without having to diet anymore. Whatever your fitness goal, becoming a "Power Positive Eater" will help you achieve what you want.

1. Do: Follow a Schedule

First, let's start with a structure or schedule to follow. I eat three small meals and three snacks each day. I don't go for longer than two or three hours without eating something. It may sound like a lot to schedule your eating. That's what I thought at first too. But now, following the schedule is just part of my routine and it really helps me keep focused and feel full throughout the day. This is how I approximately schedule my meals:

7:00 A.M.	Breakfast
9:30 A.M.	Snack #1
12:30 P.M.	Lunch
3:00 P.M.	Snack #2

| 6:00 P.M. | Dinner |
| 8:30 P.M. | Snack #3 |

Your schedule might look a little different depending on when you get up, go to work, and go to sleep. I know with families and work demands it's easy to get off the schedule. But the most important thing to remember about following a schedule is that you never want to go too long—more than three hours—without eating something, be it either a snack or a meal. Otherwise, when you do eat, you'll probably overeat.

Eating frequently seems to help control your appetite by preventing spikes in insulin production. When you eat a big meal, that causes your insulin or glucose level to spike really high. Then, afterward, you actually feel even hungrier. Surprisingly, by preventing these spikes, you even actually feel more full while eating less food.

Eating smaller meals and snacks throughout the day does more than just control your appetite. Research even shows that eating several small meals per day instead of two or three large ones actually lowers levels of cholesterol in your body.

Those three snacks are crucial to making the schedule work. Snacks keep you from feeling really hungry between meals and then overeating when you actually sit down for your full meal. Finding the right food to snack on can be a little tricky. Across the country Americans are consuming more and more snacks. That's the good news; at least we're snacking. The bad news is that those snacks don't make you healthier. Researchers found that we're eating more and more fattening, high-calorie snacks. I was surprised to learn that Americans eat on average each year:

- 45 bags of potato chips
- 120 pastries
- 125 bags of french fries
- 310 cans of 12-oz. soda
- 190 candy bars
- 150 slices of pizza

Wow! Now that's a lot of junk food!

To avoid those snacks, here are some tips for choosing a healthy snack. I've also added some of my favorites, the World's Fittest Man Snacks. These are my staples, ones I eat just about every day. You'll see I've included them in the meal plans later on in the book.

Tips for Choosing a Healthy Snack
- Choose a snack that will boost your blood sugar and keep it constant for the rest of the morning or afternoon.
- Processed sugar, like that contained in a candy bar, will give you a sugar spike and quick charge, but over time will result in fatigue and hunger, likely leading you to overeat.
- Combine a carbohydrate-rich food with a protein "chaser" or healthful fat like peanut butter. The carbohydrates will give your brain and body an immediate source of energy. A little protein or fat will help regulate the sugar from the carbohydrate so you feel full after eating.

Some examples are:

- peanut butter and celery
- turkey on whole-wheat crackers with mustard
- mixed fruit and low-fat cottage cheese
- grilled chicken strips dipped in salsa
- tuna salad with low-fat mayonnaise on whole-wheat crackers

2. Do: Downsize THIS!

Portion control is one of the easiest ways to cut back on the amount of food you eat. Now, I'm one of those guys who eats everything that's on his plate. When I was a kid growing up on the farm, my mother praised me and my brothers for leaving the table with a sparkling clean plate. Unfortunately, what was on my plate to begin with was more than enough food for a growing boy, and that led to some of my early weight problems. When I made the change to eat healthily, lose weight, and get fit, I made sure my plate was filled with just the proper portions, and not more than I wanted, or needed, to eat.

Most portions these day, especially when you go out to eat, have become supersized. That's the latest trend. You see supersized meals at many fast-food and regular restaurants. It's a way to get you to think you're getting more for your money. But what you're really getting is more fat and calories. Take, for example, McDonald's. When they first opened, a burger, fries, and Coke was a mere 590 calories. Except for all the saturated fat, that's not too bad in terms of calories. Today, a supersized McDonald's value meal—a quarter pounder with cheese, supersize fries, and a supersize drink—is about 1,500 calories. It's not just McDonald's. What about that popcorn you munch on during the movie? In 1957 that container held about three cups of popcorn. Now, it's supersized to sixteen cups and a whopping 800 calories. That's more calories than an average meal.

When you're following the meal plans in this book, be careful you stick to the allotted portions. It's easy to go overboard when it comes to pasta, bread, and rice. One of the tricks I use when I'm eating is to fill up my plate with a small salad (rather than putting the salad on another plate or salad bowl). That way the plate looks full without having to fill it with larger portions. Another great trick is to use smaller plates and bowls at mealtime. You can fill these up and still have half the calories compared to the old "feeding troughs" you once used.

3. Do: Water Yourself

I can't stress the importance of drinking water. Water helps digest your food and overall keeps your body functioning properly. Believe it or not, our bodies are about 75 percent water. I'm sure you've heard this before, but drinking water, at least six to eight glasses a day, fills you up. Often when you think you're hungry and reach for that bag of potato chips, your body is actually thirsty, not hungry. So, before you reach for that extra piece of food, down a glass of water. You'll be surprised how that glass of water will satiate your appetite.

Not only will water fill you up, but there's evidence to show that drinking water can actually help your body burn stored fat. Everything in the body takes place in a water environment. When you're dehydrated and don't have enough water, the fat just sits there. Simply put, water can help mobilize fat stored in your body.

There's even more good reason to drink water. Research shows that drinking lots of water and staying hydrated can be just as important to your cardiovascular system as working out and avoiding cigarettes. The study found that people who drink five or more glasses of water a day have half the risk of coronary heart disease compared to those who drink less than two glasses. But don't count cola, coffee, or alcohol as part of your daily water intake. Those drinks actually take water out of your body and can contribute to dehydration. Drinking water, on the other hand, thins out the blood, helping your heart pump blood better.

But let me be clear: A few glasses of water is not a meal or a snack. I still want you to follow the eating schedule. Don't try to substitute a glass of water for eating, with the idea that you'll be saving calories.

A trick that I use is to fill up a container or pitcher at the beginning of the day. If you're going to work, then use something that can be transported. Just keep the water bottle next to you and take small sips all day long. You'd be surprised how quickly the water will disappear. If you're at home, then fill up a special pitcher and put your name on it. This will be your special "World's Fittest You" water bottle, which no one else can use. Rather than leave it in the refrigerator, I'd suggest keeping it with you—that will stop you from going into the kitchen and being tempted to eat something. I'd also suggest carrying it around with you when you do your errands or travel in the car. You can be sure I don't go anywhere without a bottle of water.

Coffee

Coffee doesn't count as part of your six to eight glasses of water each day. Coffee actually has the opposite effect. A cup of coffee acts as a diuretic, meaning it causes your body to lose water. If you're going to drink coffee, do it in moderation. There is some research that shows a cup of coffee can give your metabolism a little boost by releasing fatty acids from fatty tissue. So, a cup of coffee a day is fine, but watch out for those fancy coffee drinks like lattes and Frappucinos. If you haven't noticed, they're loaded with calories and fat. I've seen some of these drinks with as many as six hundred calories.

Alcohol

Alcohol is a diuretic too. As with coffee I recommend moderation. A glass of wine or beer a few times a week with dinner is fine. Red wine, in moderation, has been shown to have a beneficial effect on your heart. But don't start drinking for that reason. If your goal is to really lose weight, then I suggest steering clear of alcohol as much as possible. A glass of wine has 72 calories and a bottle of beer 145 calories. A few glasses with dinner every night can add up.

4. Do: Read That Label

For the first four weeks of my "Shock Your Body" program, I'll be giving you a lot of guidance on how to develop healthy eating habits. Unfortunately, I won't be able to go into the supermarket with you and sort through all of the different food products. Let me tell it to you straight, looks are deceiving. You may see all of these wonderful words on the packaging like *fat free, light, good source of,* but unless you actually read the food label, you might not be getting the right information.

Be prepared. When you're reading labels it will probably take a little longer to shop. My friends hate shopping with me because I read every label. That's because I want to know exactly what I'm putting into my body. Over time it will become easier as you get used to all the different terms and numbers.

There's a lot of information on the label. Some of it is more important than others. As you become a "Power Positive Eater," these are the most important things I want you to look at closely:

- Serving Size: The serving size is how much you eat. Be careful. The serving size on the label is not necessarily what you really eat. And whatever the serving size, all the nutrition information on the label is based on one serving. If the serving size is one cup, like on the label here, and you eat two cups, then do the math. You're going to double the amount of calories and other nutrients given on the label.

Nutrition Facts

Serving Size 1 cup (228g)
Servings Per Container 2

Amount Per Serving

Calories 260   Calories from Fat 120

	% Daily Value*
Total Fat 13g	**20%**
Saturated Fat 5g	**25%**
Trans Fat 2g	
Cholesterol 30mg	**10%**
Sodium 660mg	**28%**
Total Carbohydrate 31g	**10%**
Dietary Fiber 0g	**0%**
Sugars 5g	
Protein 5g	

Vitamin A 4%	•	Vitamin C 2%
Calcium 15%	•	Iron 4%

* Percent Daily Values are based on a 2,000 calorie diet. Your Daily Values may be higher or lower depending on your calorie needs:

		Calories:	2,000	2,500
Total Fat	Less than		65g	80g
Sat Fat	Less than		20g	25g
Cholesterol	Less than		300mg	300mg
Sodium	Less than		2,400mg	2,400mg
Total Carbohydrate			300g	375g
Dietary Fiber			25g	30g

Calories per gram:
Fat 9   •   Carbohydrate 4   •   Protein 4

Source: FDA

- Calories: The total number of calories in one serving is important. Next to calories is "Calories from Fat." This tells you what part of the total calories is from fat. You want to look for foods in which the "Calories from Fat" are low, relative to the "Calories." On this label, 120 calories are from fat out of a total of 260 calories.
- Fat: The "Total Fat" includes unsaturated ("good") fat and saturated and trans ("bad") fats. Directly below "Total Fat" is often a breakdown of the types of fat in the food. Sometimes the label

breaks down the fat type, sometimes not. If there's a breakdown, as I've said before, you want to choose foods with unsaturated fat rather than saturated and trans fat. On this label, to figure out the total amount of unsaturated fat you'll have to do a little math. Add up the "Saturated Fat" and the "Trans Fat." Then, subtract that amount from the "Total Fat" and you'll get the amount of "Unsaturated Fat." In this case, the amount of unsaturated fat is 6 g. The most common source of trans fat is partially hydrogenated vegetable oil. Again, you should avoid foods with any amount of trans fat.

- Sodium: Eating too much sodium, more commonly known as salt, increases your chances of getting high blood pressure or heart disease. Look for foods that have less than 140 g per serving. That's considered "low-sodium."

- Fiber: Remember how I've said that fiber fills you up. When you look at a label, especially for a high-carbohydrate food like bread or cereal, make sure that there's some "Dietary Fiber." The more, the better. According to this label, there is no fiber. Not good. A high-fiber serving is considered five grams per serving. It's recommended you get about twenty grams of fiber total each day.

5. Do: Give Your Refrigerator a Makeover

Look in your refrigerator and take this little quiz.

- ❏ In the door I see: _____
- ❏ On the shelves I see: _____
- ❏ In the freezer I see: _____
- ❏ In the meat bin I see: _____
- ❏ In the fruit and vegetable bin I see: _____

My clients always tell me they wish they could just put a lock on the refrigerator and hide the key. They say that would make things so easy. Unfortunately, that's not a very positive approach to eating. It isn't too feasible either. That said, there are some simple and easy things to do to make your refrigerator less of a danger zone. Start by getting rid of all the tempting food that will take you off my program. Toss the whipped cream and the leftover chocolate cake. Anything that's high in saturated fat and low in nutritional value should go.

Now that all the bad stuff is gone, you're ready to give your refrigerator a much-needed makeover. Out of sight, out of mind, is what I always say. Make sure anything that's going to tempt you to eat when you open the refrigerator door is out of your direct line of sight. Like real estate it's all about location, location, location. Put it in the bottom or the back of the refrigerator. Here are some other tips:

- Position your drinking-water bottle front and center so you're always reminded to drink up.
- Place your fruits and vegetables in the front where you can see them, not down in the vegetable bin.
- Freeze leftovers or put them in the back in tightly sealed packages so you won't be tempted to nibble.
- Never eat standing in front of your refrigerator.
- If you have kids, have them hide the goodies from you.

6. Do: Substitute the Good for the Bad

Since you'll be making small changes in how you eat, it is important that you have alternatives to the food you'll be giving up. You'll be surprised by some of the healthy substitutions you can make without sacrificing taste and flavor. These foods will be not only lower in calories and fat than the "bad" foods you're eating, but they'll be loaded with fiber. When I point out some of these simple substitutions to my clients, they can't believe how easy it is. Most of the time they tell me they don't even miss the foods they're giving up, because the substitutes are even tastier. I know it may be tough cutting back on the chicken wings and beer in the beginning, but think how rewarding it will be to look down and see your old friends, your feet, again.

Take Marcy, for instance. She told me she couldn't give up her buttered bagel for breakfast each morning. I suggested two simple substitutions to cut out the fat and white flour. White bread is a high-glycemic-index food. First, I said get rid of that butter—and all that saturated fat. Instead, I suggested an all-natural jam or a thin spread of peanut butter. And instead of the bagel, two slices of whole-wheat or multigrain bread. Here are some of my favorite food substitutions. After a while you won't even notice what you're missing.

If you eat that:	Try this:
Butter	All-natural fruit preserve, jam, or jelly
Whole milk	Skim milk
Hamburgers	Chicken, turkey, tuna
Mayonnaise	Mustard or ketchup
Candy bars	Fruit
Potato chips	Carrot or celery sticks
Fried fish	Broiled, grilled, or baked fish
Hot dogs	Turkey dogs
Eggs	Egg whites or egg beaters
Sweetened cereal	Bran or fiber cereal with added fruit for taste

7. Do: Keep Track of Your Emotion Triggers

If you're like me, eating is sometimes more about how you feel than about how hungry you actually are. Certain moods, emotions, and feelings can trigger when and what you eat. Stress is one of the biggest emotional triggers. When you're stressed out it's easy to just down a cookie or candy bar. Depression is another emotional trigger. For me the depression that followed my football accident was a huge trigger to overeat. It was no problem for me to eat a large pizza, bread sticks, and a two-liter bottle of soda at one sitting. I didn't know better at the time, but I was using food to comfort and ease the emotional pain of losing my chance at a college scholarship. So the first thing is to find out if your emotions trigger you to eat:

Do I eat to comfort myself?	Yes	No
Do I eat due to boredom or loneliness?	Yes	No
Do I eat due to problems in my life?	Yes	No
Do I eat due to missing something?	Yes	No

If you answered yes to some of these questions, then you probably use food to help cope with intense emotions and feelings. To find out what some of your emotional triggers are, I recommend you keep a "World's Fittest You" eating log. Before starting my program, take a few days to record what you eat and how you feel. Keep the log in a small notebook that you can carry with you. Afterward, evaluate what emotions and feelings triggered you to overeat. If you know what the triggers are to begin with, it will ultimately be easier to control them.

WORLD'S FITTEST YOU EATING LOG

Food/Drink	How Much	Time	Where	Alone or with Whom	Activity While Eating	Mood

8. Do: Take Control

Taking control means that you're thinking about what you eat all the time. At first that's going to be hard work, I know. But soon, after you're familiar with my program, eating healthily will just become part of your normal lifestyle. For me it's hardest to "take control" when I'm eating out. When I'm home, at least I can control what I'm going to eat and how I'm going to prepare the food. The biggest pitfalls come when you're outside your own home and kitchen. Before I became the World's Fittest Man, those spicy chicken wings I'd order at restaurants were my favorite. To be honest, I could polish off fifty or sixty in one sitting. And wash it down with a few beers. Enough calories for three days. I still like to go out for dinner, but instead I'll have a roast or grilled chicken with salad and a tasty vegetable like broccoli.

The facts about eating out are telling. More and more people are eating their meals away from home. That wouldn't be so bad except that restaurant meals generally contain more fat, more calories, more cholesterol, and less fiber than homemade meals. To be sure, a restaurant meal averages twenty more grams of fat and many more calories than a home-cooked meal.

Despite these alarming statistics dining out doesn't have to be a recipe for disaster. As long as you "take control" of what you order and eat, dining out can be a positive eating experience. These are my basic tips to "take control" when you eat out. I swear by them, so you should try them too:

Taking Restaurant Control

- Speak up . . . tell the waiter how you want your food prepared.
- If there's bread on the table, send it back.
- Order appetizers as your main meal if you're worried about huge portions.
- Have a snack before dinner.
- Order a salad first with dressing on the side, so you're always eating.
- Substitute and don't be afraid to ask the waiter about this. Try a baked potato for fries, egg whites for whole eggs, garden salad or pickle instead of cole slaw.

- Get it on the side: dressing, sauces, and gravy usually have lots of calories and fats.
- Beware of buffets and salad bars—it's an invitation to overeat.
- Watch out for these words on the menu; they usually signal lots of calories and saturated fat: *butter sauce, fried, crispy, creamed, in cream sauce, au gratin, escalloped, hollandaise, béarnaise, marinated, and pastry crust.*

Some problem foods are easy to spot on a menu. You know that fried chicken or fried fish is going to be high in fat and calories. But it gets more difficult when it comes to ethnic restaurants. There, "bad" choices are harder to spot because the food is often described in a foreign language. To help in the translation, here are some words and phrases to look for to help you make healthy choices:

Chinese

steamed; jum (poached); chu (boiled); kow (roasted); shu (barbecued); hoison sauce; lightly stir-fried with light sauce; moo shu vegetable, chicken, or shrimp; chicken without skin; lean beef; lychee; wonton soup

French

vegetables; salads; crusty bread (no butter); fish, shrimp, or scallops without sauces; noodles and rice without cream sauce and butter

Italian

pasta (preferably whole wheat); lightly sautéed in olive oil; red clam sauce; piccata (lemon); grilled fish or vegetables; primavera (no cream sauce)

Middle Eastern

lemon dressing; whole-wheat pita; chick-peas; tzatkiki (yogurt and cucumbers), couscous; bulgur; lean meat grilled on a skewer, charcoal broiled, or basted in tomato sauce; plaki (fish cooked in tomatoes, onions, and garlic)

Japanese
house salad with fresh ginger; nabemono (boiled); yakimono (broiled); chicken, fish, or shrimp teriyaki; sushi or sashimi; buckwheat soba noodles

Indian
chapati (baked bread); cooked with or marinated in yogurt; tikka (pan roasted with mild spices); tandoori (marinated and oven baked); chick-peas and potatoes; chicken or shrimp kebab; paneer

Mexican
rice (preferably brown) and black beans; salsa and salsa verde; soft corn or whole-wheat tortilla; picante sauce; ceviche (marinated in lime juice and mixed with spices); chicken fajitas topped with shredded lettuce, tomatoes, and onions

Thai
chicken or fish barbecued, broiled, steamed, or marinated; basil sauce; pad thai noodles; lime sauce; Thai spices

When you're eating out at more familiar places like the local deli or a fast-food restaurant, you still have to "take control." But just as with ethnic restaurants, you should learn to order according to the "Power of Positive Eating" plan.

Taking Deli Control
- a cup of bean soup (lentil, split pea, or minestrone)
- a turkey breast, lean ham, or chicken breast sandwich with mustard and lots of vegetables on whole-wheat bread
- a fruit salad or vegetable salad with dressing on the side
- pretzels

Taking Pizza Control

- less cheese, low-fat cheese, or no cheese on your pizza
- a pizza with lots of vegetables and half the cheese
- a "salad" pizza
- chicken or ham as a topping rather than pepperoni or sausage
- whole-wheat crust

Taking Fast-Food Control

- a grilled chicken breast sandwich without mayo or cheese
- a single hamburger without cheese
- a grilled chicken salad or garden salad with low-fat or fat-free dressing on the side
- a fat-free muffin
- a veggie burger
- a baked potato with butter and toppings on the side

9. Do: Plan Ahead

This may surprise you, but a kitchen without food is a fattening one. Keep it filled. You might have thought the opposite is true—that if your kitchen is filled with food, you're more likely to overeat. From my experience it's not. I remember times when I'd open the refrigerator and there would be nothing there except some condiments and moldy bread. That's when I did the most damage to my body. Without any healthy food in the house I'd end up ordering a pizza or maybe driving down to the local convenience store to get junk food.

To keep your kitchen filled with healthy food, on my program you'll try to plan your meals a week in advance. At the beginning of each of the four weeks, look to see what foods you need to make all the meals for that week. That's how I do it, and it really works. "Planning Ahead" becomes a Sunday-night ritual for me. Here's what I do: Every Sunday night I go through my refrigerator and pantry, taking inventory of what I have and what I need. I'm very meticulous about it. I write out a big shopping list, then head out to the supermarket. Believe it or not, this method will save you time and energy. When you have everything you need in your refrigerator, it's going to make it that much easier to stick with my meal plans. Do not go to the store hungry; you will buy anything that looks good.

10. Do: Reward Yourself

I saved the best for last. This is one that I really swear by—giving yourself a reward for sticking to your healthy eating plan. For me Sunday is the day when I give myself a little treat. If Sunday doesn't work, pick a day that suits your schedule and stick with it. It's only one meal, but I treat myself to a food I've been thinking about, but not eating, all week. When I get tempted to buy that pepperoni pizza or chocolate-filled donut during the week, I say to myself, "Joe, you can have that ice cream cone, just not today, only on Sunday." Knowing that the food is not completely forbidden, and that I can indulge myself later, really takes the pressure off. I hear from so many people that they get fed up with the "don'ts" of dieting and just give up completely. This little trick gets you around all those negative dieting thoughts. Yes, I can have that scrumptious dessert, but only at my free meal on Sunday. Many of my clients tell me that after a while, they don't even crave the "free meal' and would rather just eat a healthy one. I've found that when you've worked so hard during the week, many times you don't want to even damage it on that one day.

MY FAVORITES:
THE WORLD'S FITTEST MAN'S TEN FITTEST FOODS

Joe, if you don't take a lot of supplements and pills, what do you eat to stay fit? That's one of the most common questions I get asked. For the record, these are my top ten food picks:

1. Bananas

Bananas are one of my favorite fruits. My kitchen is always stocked with a big bunch of this tropical fruit. What's great is that bananas last awhile in your kitchen and make nice ready-to-eat snacks—just peel away. As snacks, bananas are the perfect food right before or after your workout. They are a good source of potassium, which helps to control your blood pressure, and are high in vitamin B_6 to fight infection. Bananas also help your body synthesize iron for healthy blood and contain vitamin C to boost your immune system. I like bananas, too, because they have a good amount of fiber, which not only fills you up but also helps prevent diarrhea and constipation.

2. Skim Milk

Growing up on a farm, our family always had lots of milk around. What contributed to some of my early weight problems was that most of the milk I drank was very high in fat. We milked our own cows and many times would have to scrape a layer of cream off the milk jug. Now I drink skim milk almost exclusively, and usually have at least one glass each day. Skim milk is low in fat and cholesterol and at the same time it provides a good balance of protein and carbohydrates. It has vitamin A and zinc to boost your immunity, calcium to help maintain strong bones, and B_{12} for healthy nerves and blood. Some research even shows that skim milk may actually lower cholesterol, lower blood pressure, and prevent certain types of cancer.

3. Oatmeal

If you're looking for a quick, delicious breakfast food, you can't do any better than oatmeal. For my breakfast I like to spice oatmeal up with some fresh fruit like blueberries or strawberries and maybe even a little skim milk. A meal like this will really fill you up. The health benefits of oatmeal are enormous and proven through lots of scientific research. Oatmeal cuts the production of harmful cholesterol (LDL) and increases the good cholesterol (HDL). It's chockful of good vitamins and minerals like B, E, zinc, thiamine, iron, and magnesium.

4. Multigrain Bread

Bread is a great carbohydrate as long as you pick one that's high in fiber and low in calories. That's why I rely on a multigrain bread, because it's loaded with whole-grain fiber that will really fill you up. My favorite is a seven- or nine-grain type (usually available at your local supermarket). Whatever kind you choose, multigrain bread is loaded with magnesium, iron, manganese, zinc, and chromium, which help maintain strong bones.

5. Chicken

Chicken breast is one of the best sources of lean, low-fat protein. It has less fat than steak, hamburger, and many other red meats. When I prepare chicken, I usually use the breast meat and trim off all the fatty skin. Later on I'll show you some low-calorie, high-flavor recipes with chicken that I prepare all the time, like my Super Stir-fry with Chicken and Fabulous Chicken Fajitas. Chicken is also a good source of niacin, iron, and many of the B vitamins.

6. Black Beans

Black beans are the perfect food for weight loss. They're filled with lots of fiber—fourteen grams per cup. All that fiber slows your digestion and can even suppress your appetite for hours after your meal by giving you that nice full feeling. It's best to eat black beans with brown rice or some other grain so that the beans become a complete protein. If you're pressed for time, you can just open a can of black beans, saving hours of soaking time. Canned beans are just as nutritious as dry ones; just check the label on the can to make sure there's little or no added sodium. In addition to all that fiber, black beans have iron, folate, and B vitamins.

7. Cauliflower

Don't let the white color of cauliflower scare you off. It may not be as colorful as some of the other vegetables, but it sure is full of nutrients and fiber. Next to broccoli I most love to cook with cauliflower. And unlike other vegetables, cauliflower doesn't lose a lot of its nutrients when cooked. It's also one of the cancer-fighting vegetables high in vitamin C. Cauliflower can help fight infection, absorb iron into your blood, and prevent anemia.

8. Grapes

When I get that sweet-tooth craving, I love to reach for a bunch of red or green grapes. Either color will do. You'll find that the sweetness in grapes is a great substitute for a candy bar or cookie. What makes grapes so good for you is they're cholesterol free and low in sodium, fat, and calories. They even have some fiber and vitamin C. A newly discovered compound in grapes called pterostilbene seems to show promise in fighting cancer and diabetes. USDA studies have found that this compound may help protect cells from the damaging effects of carcinogens and keeps blood sugar levels under control.

9. Broccoli

I consider broccoli to be "the World's Fittest Vegetable." It can be used in so many different ways. I like it raw in salads, steamed with lemon and ginger, and sautéed with garlic and a little olive oil. One of the "Fittest" things about broccoli is that study after study has shown that it can actually help prevent cancer. What's more, it's a good source of fiber and low in calories—only fifty for a cooked cup. Broccoli is a great source of vitamin A for strong bones, teeth, and skin.

10. Tuna

Like broccoli, tuna is definitely a "World's Fittest Protein." Whether you choose canned or fresh, tuna is a perfect source of lean protein. Canned tuna is great, too, because it's relatively inexpensive. But when you buy canned tuna, make sure it's packed in water, not oil. The oil can add almost a hundred calories and fifteen grams of fat to your meal. Fresh tuna is more flavorful, but you'll end up spending quite a bit more. Both canned and fresh contain omega-3 fats, which I told you about earlier. Studies have shown that omega-3 fats decrease the risk of coronary artery disease, keep your blood sugar stable, increase your brain/mental functioning, and reduce LDL ("bad") cholesterol and raise HDL ("good") cholesterol.

EATING AND WORKING OUT

Before

I always eat a little something before a workout. Research shows that a small meal or snack eaten shortly before a workout might actually provide your body with the extra nutrients it needs to recover afterward. Those nutrients will also keep your body from using muscle protein as fuel. However, if you drink a huge shake or eat a big meal beforehand, then your body will spend too much time digesting it during the workout, causing your stomach to feel queasy.

During

When you're working out for less than an hour, which will be all of the workouts in my program (unless, of course, you're training for a competition), you don't have to worry about eating during your workout. I generally don't eat much or use sports drinks during a workout unless it's a long endurance event lasting a couple of hours. Since your workouts are going to be under an hour, all you need to do is drink lots of water. The standard is about eight to ten ounces of water every fifteen minutes during moderate-intensity exercise. You don't need to spend money on special workout drinks—water is just fine.

After

After your workout you might want another little snack if you're famished, but don't overdo it. Just because you've burned off calories, don't blow it by eating a huge meal, wasting all that hard work in the gym. If it's not time for a meal according to the schedule you're following, just have one of the prescribed snacks.

PUTTING IT ALL TOGETHER—PLANNING YOUR MEALS

Now that you understand my "Power of Positive Eating" plan and the World's Fittest You Food Guide, it's time to combine everything together. I asked nutritionist Heather Greenbaum of Nu-train to design a four-week eating plan. Nu-train is a nutrition training service based in New York City. Her company offers a highly innovative approach to weight management and sports nutrition that prescribes a combination of healthy eating and lifestyle changes. Based on this winning nutritional philosophy you'll see that for each day Heather has planned three delicious snacks and three meals for you. She's also customized the plan with two different options, depending on your specific fitness goal.

The "Weight Control" option is for those of you whose main goal is to eat healthier, become leaner and fitter, and maybe shed a few pounds. Although you don't need to count calories, if you choose this option you'll be consuming about 2,200 calories a day. The "Weight Loss" option is for those of you whose main goal is to lose weight and really shed more than a few pounds. The total number of calories you'll be consuming is 1,400. The meal plans are essentially the same as the "Weight Control" option, you'll just be decreasing some of the portion sizes and a few of the extras.

Whatever your goal, over the course of my program you'll be eating healthier to build a better body. Let the meal plans be your guide to healthy eating. I know there will probably be some foods you don't like or some you may be allergic to. That's okay. Feel free to substitute and mix and match. I've also tried to make sure the meals are easy to prepare and as simple as possible. If you're like me, the last thing you want to do after a busy day is prepare a complicated meal. Most of the meals take no more than five or ten minutes. Some of the dinners take a little bit more time, but you'll have leftovers, which you can freeze and quickly heat up later in the week and even use for lunch when you have a busy schedule. So there's no excuse for not doing it.

How did I come up with the meals? They're all based on what I eat every day to keep fit and stay in shape. These are meals that helped me become the World's Fittest Man, so I know they're proven to help you become the "World's Fittest You." To be sure, I'm not a fancy cook, but I do like to prepare my own meals. You'll see from the recipes that I've transformed many of the basic "unhealthy dishes" that my mom used to cook, like shepherd's pie and meat loaf, into delicious healthy alternatives.

SHOCK BASICS

INTRODUCTION

Now you're ready to begin my "Shock Your Body" program. I've tried to make everything as simple and straightforward as possible. I want this to be fun for you, but I also want you to challenge yourself along the way. We'll be applying all the principles that I've explained in the first few chapters. Remember, the FIT Equation will guide your workouts so that you constantly change things up and continually "Shock Your Body" for maximum results. The meal plans for each day apply the principles of my "Power of Positive Eating" program, showing you how easy it is to be healthy without having too many restrictions.

Remember, this is the "basics" week. Whether you're new to working out or not, I suggest you start slowly. You'll be learning an entirely new way to train your body, so take it easy. It's important to learn my techniques first, then you can advance at your own level. This is just the first week of a lifetime of fitness. I don't want you to burn out or injure yourself after just one week.

HOW IT WORKS

Each day of the week has a workout and meal plan. I suggest you start on a Monday so you're fresh and ready to get to work. You'll see that each day has a specific workout. Keep track of what you do that day, checking off as you go along. Each day also has what you'll be eating—the meal plan. Follow these meal plans as closely as possible. Of course you can make healthy substitutions, but I've tried to give you enough variety so that you won't get bored. You can also use my tips for eating out if you find yourself in that situation.

Even if you missed a workout day, do the "Outside the Box" workout on Saturday. This week it's my fat-blasting "Power Playground Workout." Even if you can only do a little of it, give it a try. You'll be surprised how much fun and how different it is. I can't say this enough, but one of the main reasons why people stop working out is not time, not energy, but boredom. Get family and friends involved and include as much variety as possible.

But just as you build your body, you're also going to need to rest it. Sunday is your day off. It's also your reward day for completing the week. One of your meals is what I call a "free meal." You can eat whatever you want for that meal and not feel guilty. Remember, it's only one meal and not the whole day, but this is the time to have that burger or piece of chocolate cake or fried chicken that you may have been thinking about all week. For me it's pizza and a few beers. Finally, let one of your buddies know how you did at the end of this week. Phone or e-mail them a quick update about the positive things you've accomplished. You can also e-mail me through my Web site; I'd love to hear from you.

GOALS

- Apply the principles of the FIT Equation
- Get moving five or six days this week
- Reduce saturated fat from what you eat

- Eat three small meals and three snacks each day
- Substitute multigrain or whole-grain bread for white bread
- Check out my Web site

PREPARE YOURSELF

Now that you've decided to take the next step to become "the World's Fittest You," you need to plan out how you're going to accomplish getting through this first week. If you're like me, a big factor will be time. Between working, family, and everything else in your life, you're going to have to make time for your workouts. That's all there is to it. You're going to have to work for that healthier, leaner, and stronger body. No excuses! This is for you. Ultimately your relationships, family, and work will benefit when you become happy with that person in the mirror.

No one can defeat us unless we first defeat ourselves.

—DWIGHT D. EISENHOWER

Cardio Training: 20 minutes

Activity	Frequency	Intensity	Time
	3–4 times per week	2	minutes 1–5
		4	minutes 6–15
		2	minutes 16–20

Stretch: World's Fittest Man's Total Body Stretch

FITNESS TIP: Research shows that listening to music during your workout doesn't just help you pass the time. Music can actually improve your performance, as long as the beat is fast enough. I like to listen to anything with a serious beat, from heavy metal to rap, to keep me motivated.

Breakfast   *Fittest Strawberry Oatmeal Combo:* Mix 1½ cups cooked oatmeal with 1 cup sliced strawberries and 1 cup skim milk. Serve with 1 slice of multigrain toast topped with ¼ cup whipped cottage cheese and 1 tbsp. all-natural jam.

Snack #1   1 small banana

Lunch   *Tuna Salad Pita Pocket:* Fill a six-inch whole-wheat pita with 6 oz. can of drained water-packed tuna, 1 tbsp. low-fat mayonnaise, 2 tomato slices, and ½ cup shredded lettuce.
1 apple
8 oz. low-fat yogurt
1 cup canned tomato soup

Snack #2   1 tbsp. peanut butter
8 whole-wheat crackers

Dinner   1 serving *World's Fittest Man Power Pasta Primavera* **(page 260)**

Snack #3   12 raw unsalted almonds
¼ cup raisins

1,400 Version

Breakfast   Decrease oatmeal to ½ cup; omit toast, cottage cheese, and jam

Lunch   Decrease tuna to 3 oz.; omit yogurt and soup

Snack #3   Omit raisins

FOOD TIP: Cutting down on sugar-filled soda is also an important way to cut back on calories. Here's a trick to help: Mix your soda with water, gradually increasing the amount of water over time. After a while, when you try "real" soda again, it will taste too strong and sweet.

Get Psyched: Joe's Daily Motivation

I don't believe in pessimism.

—CLINT EASTWOOD

Warm-up: 5 minutes of cardio. You choose the activity
Strength Training: Push/Ab Workout

Activity	Frequency		Weight Lbs.	Intensity	Time (minutes between sets)
	Reps	Sets			
Dumbbell bench press	12	2		2	2
Standing shoulder press	12	2		2	2
Incline dumbbell press	12	2		2	2
Front raise	12	2		2	2
Dumbbell flye	12	2		2	2
Side raise	12	2		2	2
Triceps pushdown	12	2		2	2
Triceps kickback	12	2		2	2
Parallel bar dip	12	2		2	2
Regular crunch	12	2		2	2
Reverse crunch	12	2		2	2
Elbow-to-knee crunch	12	2		2	2
Side crunch	12	2		2	2

Stretch: World's Fittest Man's Total Body Stretch

FITNESS TIP: Ever wonder about those advertisements for electrical muscle-stimulation machines that claim to get you sculpted abs, arms, and buttocks without working out? Save your money. Any fitness claims that sound too good to be true probably are. A study commissioned by the American Council on Exercise found that these machines had no effect on weight, body fat, or overall appearance. Not only that, they were painful.

Breakfast	*Fittest Cheese Omelet with Toast:* Cook 6 egg whites, 1 oz. low-fat cheese, ½ cup chopped mushrooms and tomatoes in 2 tsp. olive oil. Serve with 2 slices of multi-grain toast and 1 tbsp. all-natural jam.
Snack #1	1 pear 8 oz. skim milk
Lunch	*World's Fittest Man Turkey Sandwich:* Place 6 oz. sliced turkey breast, 1 slice avocado, and 2 cups of chopped lettuce, tomato, onions, peppers, and sprouts on 2 slices multigrain bread. Add mustard if desired. 1 cup canned minestrone soup
Snack #2	1 ½ tbsp. peanut butter 1 apple
Dinner	1 serving *World's Fittest Man Super Stir-fry with Chicken* (page 261) 1 cup cooked brown rice *Healthy Caesar Salad:* Combine 2 cups mixed greens, 2 tbsp. low-fat croutons, 2 tbsp. reduced-fat Caesar dressing. Top with 1 tsp. grated Parmesan cheese.
Snack #3	8 oz. low-fat yogurt ½ cup blueberries

1,400 Version

Breakfast	Decrease egg whites to 3 and olive oil to 1 tsp.; omit toast; substitute 1 apple for jam
Snack #1	Omit skim milk
Lunch	Decrease turkey 3 oz.; omit soup, bread, and avocado
Dinner	Omit brown rice; substitute 2 cups mixed greens tossed with balsamic vinegar for Caesar salad

FOOD TIP: Do you feel hungry right after you've eaten a meal? One way to curb your desire to snack right after a meal is to brush your teeth. That clean, fresh feeling in your mouth can help curb your cravings.

Get Psyched: Joe's Daily Motivation

> *Wake up with a smile and go after life. . . .*
> *Live it, enjoy it, taste it, smell it, feel it.*
>
> —JOE KNAPP

Cardio Training: 20 minutes

Activity	Frequency	Intensity	Time
	3–4 times per week	2	minutes 1–4
		4	minutes 5–8
		2	minutes 9–12
		4	minutes 13–16
		2	minutes 17–20

Stretch: World's Fittest Man's Total Body Stretch

FITNESS TIP: I know we're all busy, and sometimes work and family can get in the way of your workout. These are some of my favorite time-saving tips for squeezing a "mini" workout into your busy day:

- Add a ten-minute brisk walk or jog to your morning routine of picking up the paper in front of your house.
- While cooking dinner, do a few push-ups or incline push-ups (pages 214–215) against the kitchen counter.
- While you're waiting for your doctor's appointment, your daughter's ballet class, or your son's soccer practice, take a brisk walk around the block.
- During your work breaks, walk a few sets of stairs.
- If you have a meeting or lunch out of your building, take a few extra minutes to walk there.
- Try a television commercial workout. Do crunches and jumping jacks during the sales pitch.

Day 3 • WEDNESDAY

Breakfast	*Super Raisin Bran Combo:* ¾ cup raisin bran cereal ½ cup skim milk 1 cup sliced strawberries 1 hard-boiled egg 2 tomato slices 1 slice multigrain toast
Snack #1	8 oz. low-fat yogurt ½ cup low-fat granola
Lunch	*Turkey Salad with Crushed Almonds and Soup:* Mix 6 oz. diced turkey breast, 2 cups mixed greens with broccoli and cauliflower, 6 crushed raw unsalted almonds, and 1 tbsp. low-fat dressing. Serve with 1 cup canned black bean soup.
Snack #2	*Hi-NRG Turkey Snack:* 2 oz. low-fat cheese 2 oz. sliced turkey breast 6 whole-wheat crackers 1 apple
Dinner	1 serving *World's Fittest Man Fabulous Chicken Fajitas* (page 262)
Snack #3	1 small banana 1 slice multigrain toast 1 tbsp. peanut butter

1,400 Version

Breakfast	Omit toast and tomato
Snack #1	Omit granola
Lunch	Decrease turkey to 3 oz.; omit almonds
Snack #2	Omit crackers
Snack #3	Omit toast and peanut butter

FOOD TIP: Don't think that you can compensate for bad eating habits with more time working out. You can eat a hot-fudge sundae or a box of chocolate-chip cookies in a few minutes, but it will take you several hours to burn it off with a high-intensity cardio workout. Chances are, those tasty high-calorie treats are headed right to your hips or gut. Now, is that worth it?

Get Psyched: Joe's Daily Motivation

Success is due less to ability than to zeal.

— CHARLES BUXTON

Warm-up: 5 minutes of cardio. You choose the activity.

Strength Training: Pull/Leg Workout

Activity	Frequency		Weight Lbs.	Intensity	Time (minutes between sets)
	Reps	Sets			
Dumbbell squat or leg press	12	2		2	2
Regular-grip pulldown	12	2		2	2
Straight-leg dumbbell deadlift	12	2		2	2
One-arm dumbbell rows	12	2		2	2
Leg extension	12	2		2	2
Reverse-grip pulldown	12	2		2	2
Lying leg curl	12	2		2	2
Regular dumbbell curl	12	2		2	2
One-leg dumbbell calf raise	12	2		2	2
Hammer curl	12	2		2	2
Concentration curl	12	2		2	2

Stretch: World's Fittest Man's Total Body Stretch

FITNESS TIP: Patience is a virtue, especially when it comes to muscles. Your muscles won't grow or get toned overnight, despite what you may have seen in some of those body-building supplement ads. But, by sticking with your program, over time you'll get the body you want. I guarantee it!

Day 4 • THURSDAY

Breakfast	*Eye-opener Yogurt Parfait:* Divide and layer 12 oz. low-fat yogurt, 2 cups sliced strawberries, and ½ cup low-fat granola in a tall parfait glass.
Snack #1	½ cup low-fat whipped cottage cheese 7 whole-wheat crackers 20 mini carrot sticks 2 tbsp. reduced-fat ranch dressing
Lunch	*World's Fittest Man Power Pizza:* Slice open a 6-inch whole-wheat pita. Cover with ½ cup fresh chopped tomatoes, ¼ cup chopped mushrooms, ¼ cup chopped broccoli, and 2 oz. grilled chicken strips. Top with 1 oz. low-fat cheese and bake in a toaster oven or microwave until cheese is melted. Sprinkle with oregano.
Snack #2	*Chips and Salsa:* Cut a 6-inch whole-wheat tortilla into chips and coat with 1 tsp. olive oil or 3 pumps of olive oil spray. Toast in oven. Dip chips in 1 cup salsa and ½ cup low-fat cottage cheese mixture.
Dinner	1 serving *World's Fittest Man Salmon Teriyaki* (page 264) 2 cups steamed broccoli or cauliflower 1 cup brown rice
Snack #3	2 tbsp. peanut butter 2 tbsp. raisins 5 celery sticks

1,400 Version

Breakfast	Decrease yogurt to 8 oz. and strawberries to 1 cup
Snack #1	Omit carrot sticks and dressing
Snack #2	Substitute 2 oz. chicken strips and ¼ cup salsa for entire snack
Dinner	Decrease brown rice to ½ cup and vegetables to 1 cup
Snack #3	Omit raisins

FOOD TIP: Don't be a slave to the scale. Yes, it's good to keep track of your weight and your progress, but weigh yourself once a week at the most. And don't be surprised if you're not losing as much weight as you'd like. Because you're building muscle (and muscle weighs more than fat), you may actually gain a little bit of weight on my program. Here's a classic example of what I hear: "Joe, I've lost three dress sizes but I still weigh the same!" And my response: "That's great. You should be proud."

Get Psyched: Joe's Daily Motivation

Everything's in the mind. That's where it all starts. Knowing what you want is the first step toward getting it.

—MAE WEST

Cardio Training: 20 minutes

Activity	Frequency	Intensity	Time
	3–4 times per week	2	minutes 1–5
		4	minutes 6–8
		6	minutes 9–11
		4	minutes 12–14
		6	minutes 15–17
		2	minutes 18–20

Stretch: World's Fittest Man's Total Body Stretch

FITNESS TIP: I can't stress enough the importance of doing the core strength-training activities with proper form. Read through my instructions and tips carefully a few times before doing the movement. Then, try the movement without any weights so you can nail down the perfect form. You'll really get better results if you do it right, and you won't look like some of the people I see in the gym just swinging the weights around.

Day 5 • FRIDAY

Breakfast	*Breakfast Burrito Blitz:* Coat a nonstick skillet with vegetable oil spray. Scramble 1 cup Egg Beaters. Place eggs on a 9-inch whole-wheat tortilla topped with ½ cup store-bought salsa and 2 oz. low-fat cheese. Serve with ½ cup fresh squeezed orange juice.
Snack #1	½ banana ½ cup low-fat granola 8 oz. low-fat yogurt
Lunch	*World's Fittest Man Roast Beef Sandwich:* Place 4 oz. sliced lean roast beef, 1 slice low-fat cheese, and 1 tbsp. low-fat mayonnaise on 2 slices multigrain bread. Serve with 8 oz. skim milk.
Snack #2	1 tbsp. peanut butter 6 whole-wheat crackers 1 tbsp. all-natural jam
Dinner	1 slice *World's Fittest Man Awesome Turkey Meatloaf* (page 263) *Apple Walnut Salad:* Combine 1 cup mixed greens and ½ sliced apple. Top with 7 toasted walnuts, 6 raisins, and 1 tbsp. reduced-fat salad dressing.
Snack #3	2 slices low-fat cheese 6 whole-wheat crackers

1,400 Version

Breakfast	Decrease Egg Beaters to ½ cup and salsa to ¼ cup
Snack #1	Omit granola
Lunch	Omit milk; decrease roast beef to 2 oz.; substitute mustard for mayonnaise
Snack #2	Substitute 2 cups mixed vegetables with 1 tbsp. reduced-fat ranch dressing for entire snack
Dinner	Omit walnuts and raisins from salad
Snack #3	Substitute 1 apple for crackers

FOOD TIP: Not sure what's in the food you're about to eat? You'll be surprised; that food probably has more calories than you think. If you don't know a food's nutritional value, then don't eat it. Believe it or not, I've heard this one a lot: "I didn't know that fried vegetables had a lot of calories." Nice try!

> *The secret of success is constancy to purpose.*
>
> —BENJAMIN FRANKLIN

Joe's Power Playground Workout

Equipment: Jump rope
Location: A playground
Time: 30–45 minutes (depending on fitness level)

Warm-up. • Walk briskly or jog around the perimeter of the playground for 5 minutes.

Repeat the following workout 1–2 times for beginners, 3–6 times for intermediate/advanced:

Strength Stop. • Picnic Table Dip (see "Chair Dip" on page 228). Instead of a bench or chair, use a picnic table or park bench. (Use the bench part of the table, not the table itself.) Do as many dips as you can until your muscles are fatigued.

Cardio. • Skip or walk briskly two times around the perimeter of playground.

Strength Stop. • Monkey Bar Pull-up (see "Pull-up" on page 220). If you can't pull up your weight, find a bar that's close to the ground so you can use your legs for support. Do as many pull-ups as you can until your muscles are fatigued.

Cardio. • Jump rope fifty times.

Strength Stop. • Push-up (regular or modified; see pages 214–215). Do as many as you can until your muscles are fatigued.

Cardio. • Power walk or jog 3 times around perimeter of playground.

Strength Stop. • Regular Crunch (page 242). Place your feet on a picnic table or park bench. (Again, use the bench part of the table.) Do as many as you can until your abs are fatigued.

Cardio. • Picnic Table/Bench Step-up.
Stand in front of a picnic table or park bench. (Use the bench part of the table.) Step your left leg on the bench, then follow with your right. Pause, step down with your left leg, then your right leg. Repeat for 3 minutes. Go slow at first to keep your balance. If you want a more intense workout, increase your speed.

Strength Stop. • Picnic Push-up (see "Incline Push-up" on page 215).
Instead of a bench or chair, use a picnic table to lean against. Do as many push-ups as you can until your muscles are fatigued.

Cardio. • Power skip or power walk 2 times around the perimeter of the playground. A power skip is when you bring your knees to your chest with a high knee action. This really works your quad muscles.

Cool Down. • Easy walk for 5 minutes until your heart rate slows down. Then do World's Fittest Man's Total Body Stretch.

FITNESS TIP: I know it sounds obvious, but don't forget to breathe. Concentrate on air going into your lungs and energizing your whole body. Rather than short, quick breaths, focus on long, deep inhales and slow exhales. Even when you're not working out, deep breathing can relieve daily stress and help you relax.

Day 6 • SATURDAY

Breakfast *Super Waffle Combo:*
Toast 2 oat-bran waffles and top with 1 tbsp. lite
maple syrup and ½ cup blueberries. Serve with a hard-
boiled egg and 8 oz. skim milk.

Snack #1 ½ banana
½ cup bran or high-fiber cereal
8 oz. low-fat yogurt

Lunch *Salad Niçoise:*
Combine 6 oz. drained water-packed tuna with 2 cups
chopped green beans, sliced tomatoes, and chopped red
peppers. Drizzle with 1 tsp. olive oil and balsamic vinegar. Serve with a multigrain roll.

Snack #2 *World's Fittest Man Bean Dip and Pita:*
Mash together ¼ cup drained black beans, ¼ cup
store-bought salsa, 2 tbsp. canned corn, and ¼ cup
low-fat sour cream. Serve with a 6-inch whole-wheat
pita cut into small triangles and baked until crispy.

Dinner 1 serving *World's Fittest Man Lemon Grilled Salmon
with Spicy Sweet Potato Sticks* (page 265)
1 cup steamed cauliflower or broccoli

Snack #3 2 tbsp. peanut butter
6 whole-wheat crackers
½ cup skim milk

1,400 Version

Breakfast Omit syrup and skim milk

Snack #1 Omit banana

Lunch Decrease tuna to 3 oz.; omit roll

Snack #2 Decrease black beans to ⅛ cup, salsa to ⅛ cup, corn to
1 tbsp., sour cream to 2 tbsp., and pita to ½

Snack #3 Substitute 2 oz. turkey for skim milk and peanut butter; add mustard if desired

FOOD TIP: Are you a speedy eater? Don't worry, you're not alone. Most people I see eat their meals as if they're training for a Guinness World Record challenge. To slow yourself, try eating a meal with your nondominant hand (if you normally eat with the fork in your right hand, put in your left hand or vice versa). This will help you focus on every bite you take, and by the end of the meal you may feel fuller. I try using chopsticks for more meals now. That really slows me down, but sure makes it tough to eat a steak.

> *A journey of a thousand miles must begin*
> *with a single step.*
>
> —CHINESE PROVERB

Sunday's Success Story

Susan LaPierre did it . . . so can you!

Here's her story:

Susan is a married forty-one-year-old direct-marketing executive. Her busy work schedule and business travel left her tired and out of shape. What's more, lots of on-the-road take-out meals added pounds to her waist. Fitness had never been a priority for her. Growing up, she recalls trying out for the girls' volleyball team and being laughed off the court. Over the years she had tried various fitness programs, trainers, and regimes but nothing seemed to stick. She got bored quickly with step aerobics and daily gym routines. She desperately wanted a program she could maintain to keep her weight under control and her body toned and firm.

When I first met Susan about five years ago, she could hardly even run a mile. She told me her goal was to get fit, get toned, and drop some weight. She said she liked the outdoors and working out in the morning but never thought she could run any distance. I told her we would meet at 6:00 A.M., rain or shine, three or four mornings a week. At first I remember how hard it was for Susan to jog even a mile. She started out really slow. But I kept telling her speed isn't important. You don't have to be fast, you just have to be out there getting a good workout. Gradually, I worked with Susan on increasing her endurance and distance. One mile soon turned into two. Then three. At the same time I helped her strengthen her upper body and change her eating habits.

Eventually, Susan finished a 26.2-mile marathon in Richmond, Virginia—something she'd never thought she could achieve. For five and

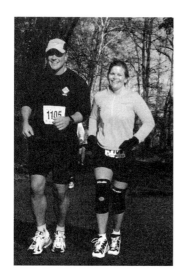

a half hours I was there by her side, telling her to just keep putting one foot in front of the other. Susan now tells me that was one of the best days of her life. It's amazing what a difference crossing that finish line has made for her. "I can do anything now," she says. "Nothing physical stops me in my tracks anymore."

Since starting my program Susan has lost fifteen pounds. Her body feels lean and strong. But more than that, Susan has integrated fitness into her life on a daily basis. And she's having *fun*. She's also helping her husband slim down. With her support he's now running two miles a day and has knocked off twenty-five pounds. Now, that's a double success!

Today's your reward day. Substitute your reward meal for one of the meals in the plan.

Breakfast *Hi-NRG Smoothie:* Blend 1 cup skim milk, 1 cup tofu, 1 cup strawberries or blueberries, and ½ cup low-fat yogurt until creamy.

Snack #1 ½ cup low-fat whipped cottage cheese
6 whole-wheat crackers

Lunch *Chicken Salad Pita Pocket and Soup:*
Fill a 6-inch whole-wheat pita with 6 oz. drained water-packed chicken breast, 1 tbsp. low-fat mayonnaise, 2 tomato slices, and 1 cup shredded lettuce. Serve with 1 cup canned lentil soup.

Snack #2 *Ants on a Log:* Cover 8 celery sticks with 2 tbsp. peanut butter. Sprinkle with 2 tbsp. raisins and serve with a sliced banana.

Dinner 1 serving *World's Fittest Man Sweet Shepherd's Pie* (page 266)

Feta Greek Salad: Mix 2 cups salad greens, ¼ cup sliced cucumber, ¼ cup sliced onions, ¼ cup sliced green peppers, and ¼ cup chopped tomatoes. Top with 1 oz. crumbled feta cheese. Drizzle with 1 tbsp. olive oil and 1 tbsp. balsamic vinegar.

Snack #3 1 apple
10 wheat crackers
2 oz. low-fat cheese

1,400 Version

Breakfast Omit tofu

Lunch Decrease chicken to 3 oz.; omit soup

Snack #2 Decrease peanut butter to 1 tbsp., banana to ½, celery sticks to 4

Dinner	Substitute 1 cup mixed green salad tossed with 1 tbsp. balsamic vinegar for Greek salad
Snack #3	Decrease apple to ½, cheese to 1 oz., crackers to 3

FOOD TIP: It's easy to overdo it on the salad dressing. Because most dressing has oil, just a small amount can add lots of extra calories to your meal. Here's a trick I use: When I'm eating out, I get dressing in a small bowl or cup. Rather than pour the dressing over the salad, dip your fork into the dressing and splash it over your salad. A splash of dressing will add flavor without all the calories. Remember, even fat-free dressing has calories. I love to make my own with balsamic vinegar, mustard, garlic, and a little olive oil. Here's my favorite dressing recipe. Simply combine the following ingredients and mix completely:

4 tbsp. balsamic vinegar

1 tsp. olive oil

½ tsp. Dijon mustard

½ tsp. garlic
salt and pepper to taste

CHAPTER 6

FEELING THE SHOCK

INTRODUCTION

You've made it through the first week. That wasn't so bad. Now you're ready for things to get a little tougher. In the first week, "Shock Basics," I introduced you to the principles of the FIT Equation. In the second week of the program you'll definitely begin "Feeling the Shock." I've added some more time to your cardio workouts. You also may want to try a new cardio activity. If you spent last week on the elliptical trainer at the gym, you may want to try the stationary bicycle for a change of pace this week. If you spent last week power walking, then maybe add a day of slow jumping rope or stair climbing. I really want you to get in the habit of changing things up and not doing the same workouts over and over again. That's why I see so many people quit. I've also added another strength-training day in place of a cardio workout. The FIT Equation variables for your strength activities are a little different too. So you'll feel your body working differently. If ever you're "Feeling the Shock" too much during this week, simply slow down or stop the activity. Remember, this is about becoming "the World's Fittest You," so you're not competing against anyone but yourself.

GOALS

- Continue to apply the FIT Equation to your workouts.
- Drink at least six to eight glasses of water per day.
- Cut out one alcoholic beverage per week.
- Add one new cardio activity to your workout, something new you may have never tried.
- Increase the time of your cardio workouts.
- Add another Push/Ab Workout to your weekly schedule.
- Write me an e-mail about your progress.

MONDAY • DAY 8

Get Psyched: Joe's Daily Motivation

The only things you regret are the things you didn't do.

—MICHAEL CURTIZ

Warm-up: 5 minutes of cardio. You choose the activity.
Strength Training: Push/Ab Workout

Activity	Frequency		Weight Lbs.	Intensity	Time (minutes between sets)
	Reps	Sets			
Dumbbell bench press	10	3		2	1
Standing shoulder press	10	3		2	1
Incline dumbbell press	10	3		2	1
Front raise	10	3		2	1
Dumbbell flye	10	3		2	1
Side raise	10	3		2	1
Triceps pushdown	10	3		2	1
Triceps kickback	10	3		2	1
Parallel bar dip	10	3		2	1
Regular crunch	10	3		2	1
Reverse crunch	10	3		2	1
Elbow-to-knee crunch	10	3		2	1
Side crunch	10	3		2	1

Stretch: World's Fittest Man's Total Body Stretch

FITNESS TIP: Want to give your walking workout a boost? Try wearing a backpack filled with a few heavy books or water bottles. Or choose a hillier course. The added weight or elevation gain can help you burn more calories.

Day 8 • MONDAY

Breakfast	*Breakfast Burrito Blitz* (page 105)
Snack #1	8 oz. skim milk
Lunch	*World's Fittest Man Turkey Sandwich* (page 99) 1 cup grapes
Snack #2	2 oz. drained water-packed tuna mixed with 1 tbsp. low-fat mayonnaise 1 oz. low-fat cheese 6 whole-wheat crackers
Dinner	1 serving *World's Fittest Man Dijon Mustard Chicken Nuggets* (page 267) 2 cups steamed broccoli and cauliflower 1 small baked sweet potato
Snack #3	8 oz. low-fat yogurt 2 tbsp. raisins ½ cup low-fat granola

1,400 Version

Breakfast	Decrease Egg Beaters to ½ cup and salsa to ¼ cup
Snack #1	Decrease skim milk to 4 oz. cup
Lunch	Decrease turkey to 3 oz.; omit bread and avocado
Snack #2	Substitute 1 cup mixed vegetables with 1 tbsp. reduced-fat ranch dressing for entire snack
Dinner	Decrease vegetables to ½ cup; omit sweet potato
Snack #3	Substitute 6 whole-wheat crackers, 1 oz. low-fat cheese, and 1 apple for entire snack

FOOD TIP: Blueberries are a great addition to your breakfast or snack. Research shows that blueberries, compared with other fruits, have the highest amount of cancer-fighting compounds called antioxidants. Blueberries are also believed to help improve your short-term memory and your balance and coordination. They are a great addition to your oatmeal too.

Get Psyched: Joe's Daily Motivation

Yard by yard, it's very hard. But inch by inch, it's a cinch.

—ANONYMOUS

Cardio Training: 25 minutes

Activity	**F**requency	**I**ntensity	**T**ime
	2–3 times per week	2	minutes 1–5
		4	minutes 6–20
		2	minutes 21–25

Stretch: World's Fittest Man's Total Body Stretch

FITNESS TIP: Don't let your baby or small child stop you from getting in your workout. Try a "baby jogger" so that you can walk or run with your little one snuggled comfortably into one of these workout-friendly strollers. You may even look for special "stroller workouts" in your local area. A friend of mine uses a "baby backpack" and even does pull-ups with his daughter on his back. Now, that's what I call giving your child a lift.

Day 9 • TUESDAY

Breakfast	*Super Raisin Bran Combo* (page 101)
Snack #1	8 oz. low-fat yogurt 1 banana ½ cup blueberries
Lunch	*World's Fittest Man Power Pizza* (page 103)
Snack #2	1 apple 2 tbsp. peanut butter 6 whole-wheat crackers
Dinner	1 serving *World's Fittest Man Paella with Brown Rice* (**page 268**) *Apple Walnut Salad* (page 105) ½ cup steamed broccoli
Snack #3	½ cup low-fat cottage cheese 1 tbsp. all-natural jam 10 whole-wheat crackers

1,400 Version

Breakfast	Omit toast and tomato
Snack #1	Omit yogurt and blueberries
Snack #2	Decrease peanut butter to 1 tbsp.
Dinner	Omit broccoli; omit walnuts and raisins from salad
Snack #3	Omit jam and crackers

FOOD TIP: Boredom can be one of those emotional triggers that may cause you to overeat. I keep lots of fruits and vegetables readily available in case boredom kicks in. Try to avoid having cookies and candy around the house, because these are sure boredom picks. I always tell myself, *If it's not there, I can't eat it.*

Get Psyched: Joe's Daily Motivation

What we prepare for is what we shall get.

—WILLIAM GRAHAM SUMNER

Warm-up: 5 minutes of cardio. You choose the activity.

Strength Training: Pull/Leg Workout

Activity	Frequency		Weight Lbs.	Intensity	Time (minutes between sets)
	Reps	Sets			
Dumbbell squat or leg press	10	3		2	1
Regular-grip pulldown	10	3		2	1
Straight-leg dumbbell deadlift	10	3		2	1
One-arm dumbbell row	10	3		2	1
Leg extension	10	3		2	1
Reverse-grip pulldown	10	3		2	1
Lying leg curl	10	3		2	1
Regular dumbbell curl	10	3		2	1
One-leg dumbbell calf raise	10	3		2	1
Hammer curl	10	3		2	1
Concentration curl	10	3		2	1

Stretch: World's Fittest Man's Total Body Stretch

FITNESS TIP: It's okay to increase the amount of weight you lift, but do it slowly. You don't want to sacrifice your good form just to show off at the gym. Using too much weight can also strain and even injure your muscles. Trust me, I know from firsthand experience.

Day 10 • WEDNESDAY

Breakfast	*Fittest Cheese Omelet with Toast* (page 99)
Snack #1	8 oz. low-fat yogurt ½ cup blueberries
Lunch	*World's Fittest Man Turkey Sandwich* (page 99) 1 cup canned lentil soup
Snack #2	*World's Fittest Man Bean Dip and Pita* (page 108)
Dinner	1 serving *World's Fittest Man White Bean Salmon Cakes* (page 270) ½ cup cooked brown rice 1 cup steamed asparagus
Snack #3	1 apple ½ cup skim milk

1,400 Version

Breakfast	Decrease egg whites to 3 and olive oil to 1 tsp.; omit toast; substitute 1 apple for jam
Lunch	Decrease turkey to 3 oz.; omit bread and avocado
Snack #2	Decrease black beans to ⅛ cup, salsa to ⅛ cup, corn to 1 tbsp., sour cream to 2 tbsp., and pita to ½
Dinner	Omit brown rice
Snack #3	Omit skim milk

FOOD TIP: It's time to say good-bye to TV dinners. If you like to eat while watching television or reading a book, think again. Research shows that eating without distractions, and focusing on your food may actually help you eat less. Think about the times you've sat down with that large pizza to watch the football game or figure skating only to realize an hour later that you just "inhaled" the whole pizza. And don't try blaming this one on your dog.

> *Knock the t off the* can't.
>
> —GEORGE REEVES

Cardio Training: 25 minutes

Activity	Frequency	Intensity	Time
	2–3 times per week	2	minutes 1–5
		4	minutes 6–10
		2	minutes 11–15
		4	minutes 16–20
		2	minutes 21–25

Stretch: World's Fittest Man's Total Body Stretch

FITNESS TIP: If something isn't scheduled in my appointment book, then chances are I'm not going to do it. That goes for working out too. To make sure I fit my workouts into my busy schedule, I write it down and schedule a time with myself. I treat this like any other important meeting. I suggest you do the same. At the beginning of each week, sit down and really schedule a specific time for your workouts. Also, make sure to have a "backup plan" in case your schedule gets too tight and you have to miss a "workout appointment."

Day 11 • THURSDAY

Breakfast	*Eye-opener Yogurt Parfait* (page 103)
Snack #1	¼ cup low-fat cottage cheese 1 tsp. all-natural jam 6 whole-wheat crackers
Lunch	*Tuna Salad Pita Pocket* (page 97) 1 orange 1 cup canned tomato soup
Snack #2	1 apple 1 slice multigrain toast 2 tbsp. peanut butter
Dinner	1 serving *World's Fittest Man Black Bean and Turkey Chili* (page 269) *Feta Greek Salad* (page 112)
Snack #3	1 oz. sliced turkey breast 1 slice low-fat cheese 6 whole-wheat crackers

1,400 Version

Breakfast	Decrease yogurt to 8 oz. and strawberries to 1 cup
Snack #1	Substitute 1 cup grapes for entire snack
Lunch	Decrease tuna to 3 oz.; omit soup
Snack #2	Decrease peanut butter to 1 tbsp.; omit apple
Dinner	Substitute 1 cup mixed green salad tossed with 1 tbsp. balsamic vinegar for Greek salad
Snack #3	Substitute 1 cup carrot and celery sticks with 1 tsp. reduced-fat dressing for entire snack

FOOD TIP: Pretzels can be a healthy snack, provided you don't eat the whole bag and stick to a sensible portion (a few ounces). You might even want to try whole-wheat pretzels because they have more fiber than regular ones. Be careful of those "gourmet" pretzels you sometimes find at the shopping mall or airport. Some of those "gourmet" pretzels can have a whopping 350 calories, and if you add some butter, 450.

Get Psyched: Joe's Daily Motivation

*We can accomplish almost anything within our ability
if we but think we can!*

—GEORGE MATTHEW ADAMS

Warm-up: 5 minutes of cardio. You choose the activity.
Strength Training: Push/Ab Workout

Activity	Frequency		Weight Lbs.	Intensity	Time (minutes between sets)
	Reps	Sets			
Dumbbell bench press	10	3		2	1
Standing shoulder press	10	3		2	1
Incline dumbbell press	10	3		2	1
Front raise	10	3		2	1
Dumbbell flye	10	3		2	1
Side raise	10	3		2	1
Triceps pushdown	10	3		2	1
Triceps kickback	10	3		2	1
Parallel bar dip	10	3		2	1
Regular crunch	10	3		2	1
Reverse crunch	10	3		2	1
Elbow-to-knee crunch	10	3		2	1
Side crunch	10	3		2	1

Stretch: World's Fittest Man's Total Body Stretch

FITNESS TIP: If you happen to get a cold and don't have a fever, then working out may not be such a bad thing for you. If your symptoms are above the neck like a runny nose, most doctors say it's okay to work out. If your symptoms are below the neck—like chest congestion, body aches or joint soreness—then skip it.

Day 12 • FRIDAY

Breakfast	*Fittest Strawberry Oatmeal Combo* (page 97)
Snack #1	1 cup grapes
Lunch	*Salad Niçoise* (page 108)
Snack #2	*Hi-NRG Turkey Snack* (page 101)
Dinner	1 serving *World's Fittest Man Catfish Creole* (page 271) 1 cup steamed broccoli
Snack #3	8 oz. low-fat yogurt ½ cup low-fat granola 1 cup sliced strawberries

1,400 Version

Breakfast	Decrease oatmeal to ½ cup; omit toast, cottage cheese, and jam
Lunch	Decrease tuna to 3 oz.; omit roll
Snack #2	Decrease cheese to 1 oz.; omit turkey
Dinner	Omit broccoli
Snack #3	Omit granola

FOOD TIP: You can really spice up your meals with some fresh herbs. My favorites are fresh basil and oregano, in the summertime. I like to add a few leaves of these to all my sauces and even sprinkle them over meat. A little extra flavor can go a long way.

Cardio. • Starbursts.

Squat lightly. Pushing off with both legs, explode and jump upward with both hands over your head. Do as many as you can until your muscles are fatigued.

Strength Stop. • Dumbbell Bench Press (page 211).

Do these chest presses lying on the ground instead of a bench. Do as many presses as you can until your muscles are fatigued.

Cardio. • Punch to the Sky.

Walk or jog in place. At the same time "throw" easy punches to the sky with alternating arms. Gradually increase the intensity. Do this for 5 minutes.

Strength Stop. • Elbow-to-Knee Crunch (page 243).

Do as many as you can until your abs are fatigued.

Cool Down. • Easy walk for 5 minutes until your heart rate slows down. Then do World's Fittest Man's Total Body Stretch.

FITNESS TIP: If you travel a lot like I do, then you know how difficult it is sometimes to squeeze in a workout. But traveling is no excuse for getting off your program. Bring your sneakers and workout clothing with you. And plan ahead. Book a hotel with a fitness center or near a park so you can do a morning power walk, jog, or an "Outside the Box" workout.

Day 13 • SATURDAY

Breakfast	*Super Waffle Combo* (page 108)
Snack #1	8 oz. low-fat yogurt ½ cup bran or high-fiber cereal ½ cup blueberries
Lunch	*World's Fittest Man Roast Beef Sandwich* (page 105)
Snack #2	2 tbsp. peanut butter 6 whole-wheat crackers 1 tbsp. all-natural jam
Dinner	1 serving *World's Fittest Man Awesome Turkey Meatloaf* (page 263) *Apple Walnut Salad* (page 105)
Snack #3	1 slice low-fat cheese 6 whole-wheat crackers

1,400 Version

Breakfast	Decrease oatmeal to ½ cup; omit toast, cottage cheese, and jam
Snack #1	Omit bran cereal
Lunch	Decrease roast beef to 2 oz.; substitute mustard for mayonnaise; omit milk
Snack #2	Decrease peanut butter to 1 tbsp.; omit jam
Dinner	Omit walnuts and raisins from salad
Snack #3	Substitute 1 apple for crackers

FOOD TIP: One of the easiest ways to cut out "empty" calories is to limit how much fruit juice you drink. I grew up on lots of sweetened drinks, so I know how easy it is to just reach for that glass of juice. Unless it's fresh squeezed, most of the stuff isn't even juice at all, just water and sugar. Go for a piece of fruit. Instead of just "empty" calories you get fiber and more nutrients.

> *Start by doing what's necessary, then what's possible,*
> *and suddenly you are doing the impossible.*
>
> —SAINT FRANCIS OF ASSISI

Sunday's Success Story

Rick did it . . . so can you!

Here's his story:

Rick is your typical family man. He's forty-one and married, with a young daughter. He has a great job, too, as organizational specialist with a national teacher's union. The only problem, that great job was unintentionally making him fat. Constant travel all over the country meant he was eating all of his meals on the go. One day it was fast food in California, the next day a greasy diner in Connecticut. His favorite meal, a cheeseburger, fries, and a beer, was always quick, easy, and available.

Those bad on-the-road eating habits eventually became normal and part of his lifestyle. At home his favorite snacks were potato chips dipped in sour cream and tortilla chips smothered with melted Velveeta cheese.

One day Rick had trouble buckling his belt on a brand-new suit. Surprised, he looked down and could barely see his feet. At thirty-six he had ballooned to 225 pounds and 28 percent body fat. That was the last straw, and at that moment he realized something had to change.

On my program Rick made some much-needed changes. Here's some of the ways he told me he did it:

- I made exercise the first thing I do in the morning no matter what. When you pop out of bed and do your workout, your body is on fire for the rest of the day.
- I always have a fitness goal.

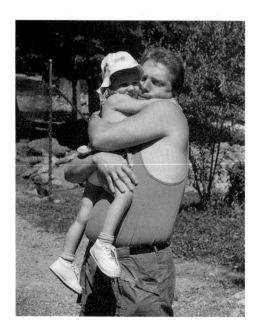
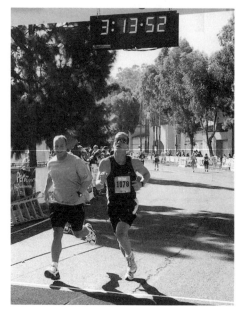

- I work out every day.
- I don't diet; I just make smart choices.
- I don't eat junk food.
- I keep a workout log because I find it very motivating to see what I've accomplished. It makes me feel guilty if there's nothing in the book.

Like it or not, Rick still travels for his job. But now, after following my program, he's able to "take control" when he eats out. Rick isn't afraid to speak up and tell the waiter exactly what he wants. When he chooses something from the menu, the first thing he asks himself is "What can I drop or substitute?" Instead of those fat-laden fries he asks for vegetables or a baked potato.

"Everything on the side" is another one of Rick's tips; salad dressing, sour cream, sauces. Even if it's fast food like Subway, he'll chose turkey over fatty cold-cut meats.

Whether he's on the road or at home, working out is now an integral part of Rick's lifestyle. To keep motivated he challenges himself with different running races and events throughout the year.

Today's your reward day. Substitute a reward meal for one of the meals in the plan.

Breakfast   *Hi-NRG Smoothie* (page 112)

Snack #1   6 whole-wheat crackers
                ½ cup low-fat cottage cheese
                1 tsp. all-natural jam

Lunch   *World's Fittest Man Power Pizza* (page 103)

Snack #2   *World's Fittest Man Bean Dip and Pita* (page 108)

Dinner   1 serving *World's Fittest Man Lemon Grilled Salmon
                with Spicy Sweet Potato Sticks* (page 265)
                1 cup steamed broccoli and cauliflower

Snack #3   6 whole-wheat crackers
                2 tbsp. peanut butter
                ½ cup skim milk

1,400 Version

Breakfast   Omit tofu

Snack #2   Decrease black beans to ⅛ cup, salsa to ⅛ cup, corn to
                1 tbsp., sour cream to 2 tbsp., and pita to ½

Dinner   Decrease vegetable mix to 1 cup

Snack #3   Substitute 2 oz. turkey for peanut butter; add mustard
                if desired

FOOD TIP: Sometimes just plain old water can be a drag, I know. Try this: Add a few slices of lemon or lime. Or throw in a few mint leaves. You can even charge it up with flavored seltzer or soda water. Just make sure the flavoring is just that, flavor, and not extra calories.

CHAPTER 7

INTENSIFYING THE SHOCK

INTRODUCTION

With two weeks of the program under your belt, you're ready to pump up the intensity a little. This week I really want you to focus on Intensity, whether you're doing cardio or strength training. By now you should be getting into a routine—planning for when you're going to work out and what you're going to eat. This week I also want you to focus on your stretching. Are you doing the Total Body Stretch after each workout or are you skipping past it? If you can't do all the stretches one day, then do half—and do the other half the next day. But you should make time for stretching at the end of your workout.

GOALS

- Increase cardio time to thirty minutes.
- Add one more cardio activity, preferably outdoors.
- Focus on the Intensity in the FIT Equation.
- Increase the amount of weight in your strength-training activities, if you can.

- Increase the hold time of your stretch by a few seconds.
- If you're doing my program at the gym, try a few of the "home-version" strength-training activities to add variety.
- Bring a friend or family member to your "Outside the Box" workout.
- If you eat out, ask your waiter to prepare your food so it's healthy and the way you want it.
- Go to my Web site and find a "World's Fittest You" buddy.

Get Psyched: Joe's Daily Motivation

> *The man who removes the mountain begins*
> *by carrying away small stones.*
>
> —CHINESE PROVERB

Cardio Training: 30 Minutes

Activity	Frequency	Intensity	Time
	3–4 times per week	2	minutes 1–5
		4	minutes 6–9
		6	minutes 10–13
		2	minutes 14–17
		4	minutes 18–21
		4	minutes 22–25
		4	minutes 26–30

Stretch: World's Fittest Man's Total Body Stretch

FITNESS TIP: Believe it or not, the abs are one of the most difficult muscles to train correctly. In order to get the best results you have to focus on feeling your abs contract more than just doing the movement itself. Don't just flop around on the ground like many people I see in the gym. Concentrate!

Day 15 • MONDAY

Breakfast	*Breakfast Burrito Blitz* (page 105)
Snack #1	8 oz. low-fat yogurt 1 cup grapes
Lunch	*Chicken Salad Pita Pocket and Soup* (page 112)
Snack #2	*Hi-NRG Turkey Snack* (page 101)
Dinner	1 serving *World's Fittest Man Fabulous Chicken Fajitas* (page 262)
Snack #3	1 banana 2 tbsp. peanut butter 6 whole-wheat crackers

1,400 Version

Breakfast	Decrease Egg Beaters to ½ cup and salsa to ¼ cup
Snack #1	Omit yogurt
Lunch	Decrease chicken to 3 oz.; omit soup
Snack #2	Decrease cheese to 1 oz.; omit turkey
Snack #3	Decrease banana to ½, substitute ½ cup skim milk for peanut butter and crackers

FOOD TIP: It's easy to use too much oil when you're cooking. Even though my recipes call for olive oil, one of the good fats, an extra tablespoon or two is hundreds of extra calories. Don't ever just pour from the bottle, always use a measuring spoon to portion out the oil. Even better, you might want to get olive oil in a spray can rather than a bottle for cooking or sautéing.

Get Psyched: Joe's Daily Motivation

It is never too late to be what you might have been.

—GEORGE ELIOT

Warm-up: 5 minutes of cardio. You choose the activity.

Strength Training: Pull/Leg Workout

Activity	Frequency		Weight Lbs.	Intensity	Time (minutes between sets)
	Reps	Sets			
Dumbbell squat or leg press	12	2		3	2
Regular-grip pulldown	12	2		3	2
Straight-leg dumbbell deadlift	12	2		3	2
One-arm dumbbell row	12	2		3	2
Leg extension	12	2		3	2
Reverse-grip pulldown	12	2		3	2
Lying leg curl	12	2		3	2
Regular dumbbell curl	12	2		3	2
One-leg dumbbell calf raise	12	2		3	2
Hammer curl	12	2		3	2
Concentration curl	12	2		3	2

Stretch: World's Fittest Man's Total Body Stretch

FITNESS TIP: Gripping dumbbells can sometimes cause you to get calluses on your hands. Some of my clients have told me that they have trouble just holding on to the dumbbell. If that's the case, don't think you're off the hook. There's a simple solution: invest in a pair of weight-training gloves. You can get a good pair for under $20. And don't think these gloves are just for those bodybuilders. I trained a sixty-two-year-old woman who used a pair of weight gloves to get a better grip. She swears by them.

Day 16 • TUESDAY

Breakfast	*Super Raisin Bran Combo* (page 101)
Snack #1	1 cup strawberries
Lunch	*World's Fittest Man Turkey Sandwich* (page 99) 1 cup canned lentil soup
Snack #2	*Ants on a Log* (page 112)
Dinner	1 serving *World's Fittest Man Dijon Mustard Chicken Nuggets* (page 267) 2 cups steamed broccoli and cauliflower mix 1 small baked sweet potato
Snack #3	6 whole-wheat crackers 1 oz. low-fat cheese 1 apple

1,400 Version

Breakfast	Omit toast and tomato
Lunch	Decrease turkey to 3 oz.; omit soup, bread, avocado
Snack #2	Decrease peanut butter to 1 tbsp., banana to ½, celery sticks to 4
Dinner	Decrease vegetables to ½ cup
Snack #3	Omit crackers and cheese

FOOD TIP: Watch out for those energy drinks and bars during your workout. Unless you're working out for more than one hour, you really don't need these supplements. They just add extra calories. An energy drink can have over 200 calories. And some energy bars have as many as 300 calories. You're better off having one of your snacks from the meal plan just after you finish working out.

Eighty percent of success is showing up.

—WOODY ALLEN

Warm-up: 5 minutes of cardio. You choose the activity.
Cardio Training: 30 minutes

Activity	Frequency	Intensity	Time
	3–4 times per week	2	minutes 1–5
		4	minutes 6–15
		2	minutes 16–20
		5	minutes 21–25
		2	minutes 26–30

Stretch: World's Fittest Man's Total Body Stretch

FITNESS TIP: It's okay once in a while to read a magazine or book during your cardio workout. But reading can sometimes distract you too much from focusing on following the FIT Equation. I see many people in the gym exercising their eyes more than their bodies. You'll get a more intense workout and burn more calories listening to high-energy music and paying attention to your body.

Day 17 • WEDNESDAY

Breakfast	*Fittest Cheese Omelet with Toast* (page 99)
Snack #1	1 banana 8 oz. skim milk
Lunch	*Salad Niçoise* (page 108)
Snack #2	½ cup low-fat whipped cottage cheese 1 cup sliced strawberries 6 whole-wheat crackers
Dinner	1 serving *World's Fittest Man Salmon Teriyaki* (page 264) 2 cups steamed broccoli 1 cup cooked brown rice
Snack #3	8 oz. low-fat yogurt ½ cup low-fat granola

1,400 Version

Breakfast	Decrease egg whites to 3 and olive oil to 1 tsp.; omit toast; substitute 1 apple for jam
Lunch	Decrease tuna to 3 oz.; omit roll
Dinner	Decrease broccoli to ½ cup and brown rice to ½ cup
Snack #3	Omit granola

FOOD TIP: Is your office refrigerator packed with your colleagues' spoiled food? Do you travel in your car and end up at the fast-food drive-thru for lunch? If so, try carrying a travel-size cooler around with you. Pack it with a few reusable ice packs and your food can stay fresh all day. This way, you can keep your healthy snacks and meals with you wherever you go.

Get Psyched: Joe's Daily Motivation

I have learned to use the word impossible
with the greatest caution.

—WERNHER VON BRAUN

Warm-up: 5 minutes of cardio. You choose the activity.

Strength Training: Push/Ab Workout

Activity	Frequency		Weight Lbs.	Intensity	Time (minutes between sets)
	Reps	Sets			
Dumbbell bench press	12	2		3	2
Standing shoulder press	12	2		3	2
Incline dumbbell press	12	2		3	2
Front raise	12	2		3	2
Dumbbell flye	12	2		3	2
Side raise	12	2		3	2
Triceps pushdown	12	2		3	2
Triceps kickback	12	2		3	2
Parallel-bar dip	12	2		3	2
Regular crunch	12	2		3	2
Reverse crunch	12	2		3	2
Elbow-to-knee crunch	12	2		3	2
Side crunch	12	2		3	2

Stretch: World's Fittest Man's Total Body

FITNESS TIP: If you want to add some variation and relaxation to your stretching routine, try a yoga class. They're so popular now that most gyms offer them. You can even find yoga classes at your local YMCA or recreation center. Make sure you start with a basic class, otherwise you might get frustrated with the movements. And for you men, yoga is not just for women. You'd be surprised how many men I've seen in yoga classes these days. It's a lot tougher than it looks, guys!

Breakfast	*Eye-opener Yogurt Parfait* (page 103)
Snack #1	1 cup grapes
Lunch	*World's Fittest Man Roast Beef Sandwich* **(page 105)**
Snack #2	2 tbsp. peanut butter 6 whole-wheat crackers 1 tbsp. all-natural jam
Dinner	1 serving *World's Fittest Man Sweet Shepherd's Pie* **(page 266)** *Feta Greek Salad* (page 112)
Snack #3	1 apple 10 whole-wheat crackers 2 oz. low-fat cheese

1,400 Version

Breakfast	Decrease yogurt to 8 oz. and strawberries to 1 cup
Lunch	Omit milk; decrease roast beef to 2 oz.; substitute mustard for mayonnaise
Snack #2	Substitute 2 cups chopped mixed vegetables with 1 tbsp. low-fat ranch dressing for entire snack
Dinner	Substitute 1 cup mixed green salad tossed with 1 tbsp. balsamic vinegar for Greek salad
Snack #3	Omit crackers

FOOD TIP: Are you having an unbelievable craving for candy or some other sugary sweet today? Don't despair! Research shows that sipping a cup of green tea may help to reduce appetite and food cravings. Green tea is also reported to raise the level of antioxidants in your blood to help ward off cancer and heart disease. Green tea does contain caffeine, so if you want to avoid it, try a brand that's decaffeinated. Keep in mind, green tea isn't a "magic bullet" for weight loss—you've got to be following your program too.

Get Psyched: Joe's Daily Motivation

The body manifests what the mind harbors.

—JERRY AUGUSTINE

Cardio Training: 30 minutes

Activity	Frequency	Intensity	Time
	3–4 times per week	2	minutes 1–6
		4	minutes 7–12
		2	minutes 13–18
		4	minutes 19–24
		2	minutes 25–30

Stretch: World's Fittest Man's Total Body Stretch

FITNESS TIP: Always lift weights in controlled and deliberate movements. Slow and steady is the name of the game. You control the weights; don't let the weights control you.

Day 19 • FRIDAY

Breakfast	*Super Waffle Combo* (page 108)
Snack #1	8 oz. low-fat yogurt ½ cup bran or high-fiber cereal ½ cup blueberries
Lunch	*World's Fittest Man Power Pizza* (page 103)
Snack #2	*Chips and Salsa* (page 103)
Dinner	1 serving *World's Fittest Man Black Bean and Turkey Chili* (page 269) *Feta Greek Salad* (page 112)
Snack #3	*Ants on a Log* (page 112)

1,400 Version

Breakfast	Omit syrup and skim milk
Snack #1	Omit cereal
Snack #2	Substitute 2 oz. chicken strips and ¼ cup salsa for entire snack
Dinner	Omit salad
Snack #3	Substitute 1 tbsp. peanut butter and 1 apple for entire snack

FOOD TIP: Do you feel that sweet tooth coming again? Keep a bowl of washed grapes, blackberries, or raspberries in the front of your refrigerator where you can see them, or near your desk at work. You can even freeze them in a Ziploc bag and munch on them like crunchy candy to satisfy that sweet craving. A few grapes are a whole lot better for you than candy.

Shoot for the moon. Even if you miss it, you will land among the stars.

—LES BROWN

Joe's Dirty Diamond Workout
Location: Baseball field
Equipment: None
Time: 30–45 minutes

Warm-up. • 5-minute brisk walk or jog around the baseball field. Repeat the following workout 1–2 times for beginners, 3–6 times for intermediate/advanced.

Cardio-Combo. • "Ballpark Push-up" (see "Push-up" on page 214). Start at home base. Jog or power walk to first base. Do as many push-ups as you can in 10 seconds. Jog or power walk to second base. Do as many push-ups as you can in 10 seconds. Jog or power walk to third base. Do as many push-ups as you can in 10 seconds. Jog or power walk back home. Do as many push-ups as you can in 10 seconds.

Strength Stop. • Dumbbell Squat (page 232). Just do the squat movement; you don't need to use any dumbbells or weights. Do as many as you can until your muscles are fatigued.

Cardio. • "Suicides." Jog or walk briskly from home plate to the pitcher's mound and back. Then, go from home plate to second base and back home. Finally, go from home plate to the outfield and then back home. Do as many Bench Dips (see "Chair Dip" page 228) as you can until your muscles are fatigued.

Cardio-Combo. • "Ballpark Crunches" (see "Regular Crunch," page 242). Start at home base. Jog or power walk to first base. Do as many crunches as you can in 30 seconds. Jog or power walk to second base. Do as many crunches as you can in 30 seconds. Jog or power walk to third base. Do as many crunches as you can in 30 seconds. Jog or power walk back home. Do as many crunches as you can in 30 seconds.

Strength Stop. • Walking Lunge (see "Dumbbell Lunge" on page 240).

Do as many as you can until your muscles are fatigued. You don't need to use any dumbbells.

Cardio. • Run up and down the bleacher steps for 5 minutes. If there are no stairs, do the Picnic Table/Bench Step-up (page 107).

Cool Down. • Easy walk for 5 minutes until your heart rate slows down. Then do World's Fittest Man's Total Body Stretch.

FITNESS TIP: Missing a workout isn't the end of the world. Just let it go and don't fret about it. Figure out why you missed it so you make sure it doesn't happen again. Most of all, don't do double-time the next day—that is, don't do twice as much to make up for what you missed. You risk straining and injuring yourself if you do. You can do this later on down the road when you've become a pro.

Day 20 • SATURDAY

Breakfast	*Fittest Strawberry Oatmeal Combo* (page 97)
Snack #1	8 oz. low-fat yogurt 12 raw unsalted almonds ¼ cup raisins
Lunch	*Tuna Salad Pita Pocket* (page 97)
Snack #2	*Hi-NRG Turkey Snack* (page 101)
Dinner	1 serving *World's Fittest Man Power Pasta Primavera* (page 260)
Snack #3	½ banana

1,400 Version

Breakfast	Decrease oatmeal to ½ cup; omit toast, cottage cheese, and jam
Snack #1	Omit yogurt
Lunch	Decrease tuna to 3 oz.
Snack #2	Decrease cheese to 1 oz.

FOOD TIP: Surprised by the peanut butter snacks in my eating plan? Don't be! Peanut butter is healthier than you may think. Research shows that a few small helpings of peanuts or peanut butter a week can help lower your risk of developing adult-onset diabetes, particularly for women. When you buy peanut butter, be sure to look at the label closely. Some kinds of peanut butter have added sugar and trans fat. Stick to the "natural" stuff that's just pure peanuts.

Get Psyched: Joe's Daily Motivation

> *We can do anything we want to do*
> *if we stick to it long enough.*
>
> —HELEN KELLER

Sunday's Success Story

Marcy did it . . . so can you!

Here's her story:

Marcy was stuck in a rut. At thirty-two and working as a computer software designer, she had gained twenty pounds. It didn't help that she was sitting in front of a computer terminal most of the day. She had worked out before but suddenly found herself unmotivated and bored with her normal workout routines. Her eating habits changed too. She was snacking on fattening treats like chocolate-chip cookies and tortilla chips.

She needed something drastic to get her excited about fitness and knock off those unwanted pounds. "The gym," she said, "just wasn't working for me." I knew just the trick: Marcy needed to start having "fitness fun." I introduced Marcy to some of my "Outside the Box" workouts—boot-camp style—to get her out of the gym and into the great outdoors. Here's what I had her doing: lifting rocks at construction sites, running up and down piles of dirt, pushing picnic tables back and forth, doing crunches with weights of timber, and dropping and rolling in the grass like a football player. Rain or shine, Marcy was out there. Some days she came home so dirty, her husband didn't even recognize her. But she loved every minute of it and suddenly found herself actually enjoying her workouts. "What you put me through was more intense than anything I did at the gym. And lots more fun," she told me.

The "Power of Positive Eating" plan also helped Marcy change her eating habits. Rather than loading up on carbohydrates like bread and pasta, she started to balance out her meals: more chicken, fish, fruit, and vegetables. I remember Marcy told me that the hardest part for her was drinking those eight glasses of water each day. For her, water was just too bland. So here's how she spiced things up: a wedge of lemon or lime to add some flavor and seltzer or sparkling water instead of just plain water.

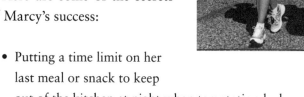

Here are some of the secrets of Marcy's success:

- Putting a time limit on her last meal or snack to keep out of the kitchen at night when temptation lurks
- Reading the food label, looking closely at fiber and fat content
- Having a fitness goal to keep motivated

Now, I am happy to report, Marcy is down to her 120-pound weight goal, has completed a marathon, and is energized and excited about continuing to work out. Her favorite reward food: a strawberry-kiwi fruit Newton.

Today's your reward day. Substitute your reward meal for one of the meals in the plan.

Breakfast   *Hi-NRG Smoothie* (page 112)

Snack #1   8 oz. low-fat yogurt
1 cup grapes

Lunch   *Chicken Salad Pita Pocket and Soup* (page 112)

Snack #2   *Hi-NRG Turkey Snack* (page 101)

Dinner   1 serving *World's Fittest Man Catfish Creole* (page 271)
1½ cups steamed broccoli

Snack #3   8 oz. low-fat yogurt
¼ cup low-fat granola
1 cup sliced strawberries

1,400 Version

Breakfast   Omit tofu

Snack #1   Omit yogurt

Lunch   Decrease chicken to 3 oz.; omit soup

Snack #2   Decrease cheese to 1 oz.; omit turkey

Dinner   Decrease broccoli to ½ cup

Snack #3   Omit granola

FOOD TIP: Every spoonful counts, including that spoonful of sugar you add to your cereal, coffee, or tea. First, see if you can do without the sweetener altogether. If not, try a no-cal sweetener like Equal or Sweet'N Low. Be careful with honey. Although it's not made from white refined sugar, it still actually has more calories per serving than sugar.

CHAPTER 8

ENJOYING THE SHOCK

INTRODUCTION

You've made it to the fourth week of the program. You should now be more comfortable with using the FIT Equation and my healthy eating plan. Things should start getting fun this week. You should start "Enjoying the Shock." You should also start to feel and see changes in your body. Notice all these changes and congratulate yourself on a job well done. Yes, this is the final week of the program, but it's also just the beginning. It's the beginning of a new you, and a new way of life. Make sure to take the fitness test at the end of the week and compare your progress.

GOALS

- Add another cardio activity to your routine, preferably something you have never tried before.
- Work out with a friend or family member one day, then cook one of the delicious dinner recipes for him or her.
- Repeat each stretch two times.
- Try a new vegetable and substitute it for one in the plan.

- Notify your "World's Fittest You" buddies that you've completed the four-week program.
- Try a few of the "Fittest Variations" when you do your strength-training activities.
- Look through the "Challenge Yourself!" chapter and start thinking about a challenge you can prepare for in the coming weeks and months.

Get Psyched: Joe's Daily Motivation

Change your thoughts and you change your world.

—NORMAN VINCENT PEALE

Warm-up: 5 minutes of cardio. You choose the activity.

Strength Training: Pull/Ab Workout

Activity	Frequency		Weight Lbs.	Intensity	Time (minutes between sets)
	Reps	Sets			
Regular-grip pulldown	10	3		3	1
One-arm dumbbell row	10	3		3	1
Reverse-grip pulldown	10	3		3	1
Regular dumbbell curl	10	3		3	1
Hammer curl	10	3		3	1
Concentration curl	10	3		3	1
Regular crunch	10	3		3	1
Reverse crunch	10	3		3	1
Elbow-to-knee crunch	10	3		3	1
Side crunch	10	3		3	1

Stretch: World's Fittest Man's Total Body Stretch

FITNESS TIP: One of the great things about working out and increasing your physical activity is that it can actually improve your sex drive. Most people think it's just the opposite, that if you work out you'll be too tired for sex. Absolutely not. As you get fit, you'll probably find your sexual desire and performance reinvigorated. And we don't even charge extra for this.

Day 22 • MONDAY

Breakfast	*Super Raisin Bran Combo* (page 101)
Snack #1	½ cup low-fat granola 8 oz. low-fat yogurt
Lunch	*Turkey Salad with Crushed Almonds and Soup* (page 101)
Snack #2	2 tbsp. peanut butter 6 whole-wheat crackers 1 tbsp. all-natural jam
Dinner	1 serving *World's Fittest Man Awesome Turkey Meatloaf* (page 263) *Apple Walnut Salad* (page 105)
Snack #3	½ cup low-fat whipped cottage cheese 6 whole-wheat crackers

1,400 Version

Breakfast	Omit toast and tomato
Snack #1	Decrease yogurt to 4 oz. and granola to ¼ cup
Lunch	Decrease turkey to 3 oz.; omit almonds
Snack #2	Substitute 2 cups mixed vegetables with 1 tbsp. reduced-fat ranch dressing for entire snack
Dinner	Omit walnuts and raisins from salad
Snack #3	Decrease cottage cheese to ¼ cup and crackers to 3

FOOD TIP: Here's an easy way to transform your everyday boring salad into a delicious and satisfying meal. Toss a few black beans (one of my Fittest Foods), chick-peas, or kidney beans into your salad to boost the fiber and nutrients, making the salad much more filling. I always keep extra cans of beans in the cupboard just for this purpose.

All that we are is the result of what we have thought. The mind is everything. What we think, we become.

— BUDDHA

Cardio Training: 35 minutes

Activity	Frequency	Intensity	Time
	2–3 times per week	2	minutes 1–5
		4	minutes 6–10
		6	minutes 11–15
		2	minutes 16–20
		4	minutes 21–25
		6	minutes 26–30
		2	minutes 31–35

Stretch: World's Fittest Man's Total Body Stretch

FITNESS TIP: Do you have a big presentation or tough exam coming up? Rather than spending all your extra time preparing and studying, take a break to work out. New research shows that forty-five minutes of physical activity can bolster your memory and improve your thinking ability. A strong body yields a strong mind.

Breakfast	*Fittest Cheese Omelet with Toast* (page 99)
Snack #1	½ cup low-fat whipped cottage cheese 6 whole-wheat crackers
Lunch	*Salad Niçoise* (page 108)
Snack #2	6 whole-wheat crackers 2 tbsp. peanut butter 1 banana
Dinner	1 serving *World's Fittest Man Fabulous Chicken Fajitas* (page 262)
Snack #3	8 oz. low-fat yogurt ¼ cup low-fat granola ½ cup blueberries

1,400 Version

Breakfast	Decrease egg whites to 3 and olive oil to 1 tsp.; omit toast; substitute 1 apple for jam
Lunch	Decrease tuna to 3 oz.; omit roll
Snack #2	Substitute 1 apple for banana, decrease peanut butter to 1 tbsp.
Snack #3	Decrease yogurt to 4 oz. and granola to 2 tbsp.

FOOD TIP: Take it from me, portion control is tough when you're eating out and more and more meals are now supersized. Here's a trick: Order something from the kids' menu. Not only are the portions smaller, but you'll even save a few bucks while you're at it. You'll most likely find yourself full but not "superstuffed" after this meal. Exactly what you want.

Get Psyched: Joe's Daily Motivation

Our destiny changes with our thoughts; we shall become what we wish to become, do what we wish to do, when our habitual thoughts correspond with our desires.

—ORISON SWETT MARDEN

Warm-up: 5 minutes of cardio. You choose the activity.

Strength Training: Push/Leg Workout

Activity	Frequency		Weight Lbs.	Intensity	Time (minutes between sets)
	Reps	Sets			
Dumbbell bench press	10	3		3	1
Standing shoulder press	10	3		3	1
Dumbbell squat or leg press	10	3		3	1
Incline dumbbell press	10	3		3	1
Leg extension	10	3		3	1
Front raise	10	3		3	1
Leg curl	10	3		3	1
Dumbbell flye	10	3		3	1
Side raise	10	3		3	1
One-leg dumbbell calf raise	10	3		3	1
Triceps pushdown	10	3		3	1
Triceps kickback	10	3		3	1
Parallel bar dip	10	3		3	1

Stretch: World's Fittest Man's Total Body Stretch

FITNESS TIP: If you're using headphones during your outdoor cardio activities, be careful. I recommend using only one earphone so that the other ear can be tuned in to your surroundings. If you're biking, I suggest you leave the headphones at home altogether.

Day 24 • WEDNESDAY

Breakfast	*Eye-opener Yogurt Parfait* (page 103)
Snack #1	6 raw unsalted almonds ¼ cup raisins 15 mini wheat pretzels
Lunch	*World's Fittest Man Power Pizza* (page 103)
Snack #2	*Chips and Salsa* (page 103)
Dinner	1 serving *World's Fittest Man Dijon Mustard Chicken Nuggets* (page 267) 2 cups steamed broccoli and cauliflower 1 small baked sweet potato
Snack #3	*Ants on a Log* (page 112)

1,400 Version

Breakfast	Decrease yogurt to 8 oz. and strawberries to 1 cup
Snack #1	Omit almonds and pretzels
Snack #2	Substitute 2 oz. of chicken strips and ¼ cup salsa for entire snack
Dinner	Decrease vegetables to ½ cup
Snack #3	Substitute 1 tbsp. peanut butter and ½ apple for entire snack

---

FOOD TIP: We're all human so it's only natural that you may slip off the eating plan once in a while. If you pig out when you're not supposed to, don't get depressed. Figure out what triggered you to slip. Was it emotional stress? Was it lack of time? Once you've done this, get back on track. Believe me, you're not alone; I've been known to slip off every now and then. Especially when it comes to pizza.

Get Psyched: Joe's Daily Motivation

You can't pay attention to your mistakes. I made a mistake today, I made a mistake yesterday. I think it's . . . very important to ignore the negative.

—JERRY RUBIN

Cardio Training: 35 minutes

Activity	Frequency	Intensity	Time
	2–3 times per week	2	minutes 1–5
		4	minutes 6–15
		6	minutes 16–25
		4	minutes 26–30
		2	minutes 31–35

Stretch: World's Fittest Man's Total Body Stretch

FITNESS TIP: Before you start your workout routine, whether it's at home or the gym, take a minute or two to visualize what you're going to do. Try to think about how much fun you're going to have and not about how big of a jerk your boss may be. Also, if you haven't done so in a while, take a moment to look back at your goals and what you're trying to accomplish. Warming up your mind with mental preparation is just as important as warming up your body before a workout.

Day 25 • THURSDAY

Breakfast	*Super Waffle Combo* (page 108)
Snack #1	¼ cup low-fat cottage cheese 1 tsp. all-natural jam 6 whole-wheat crackers
Lunch	*World's Fittest Man Roast Beef Sandwich* (page 105)
Snack #2	*World's Fittest Man Bean Dip and Pita* (page 108)
Dinner	1 serving *World's Fittest Man White Bean Salmon Cakes* (page 270) ½ cup cooked brown rice 1 cup steamed asparagus tips
Snack #3	8 oz. low-fat yogurt ½ cup bran or high-fiber cereal ½ cup blueberries

1,400 Version

Breakfast	Omit syrup and skim milk
Snack #1	Substitute 1 cup grapes for entire snack
Lunch	Omit milk; decrease roast beef to 2 oz.; substitute mustard for mayonnaise
Snack #2	Decrease black beans to ⅛ cup, salsa to ⅛ cup, corn to 1 tbsp., sour cream to 2 tbsp., and pita to ½
Dinner	Omit brown rice
Snack #3	Omit blueberries

FOOD TIP: Just as I've been saying how important it is to vary your workout, you should do the same for your healthy eating plan. I like to have a Mexican, Italian, or Oriental food night at least once a week. And I try all kinds of different fish and healthy methods of preparation. I've given you lots of meal choices and recipes in this book. But when you're looking for more variety, check out my Web site for new recipes and healthy eating options. The more options you have, the less you'll feel like you're on an awful "diet."

Get Psyched: Joe's Daily Motivation

*Optimism is essential to achievement and is also
the foundation of courage and of true progress.*

—NICHOLAS MURRAY BUTLER

Warm-up: 5 minutes of cardio. You choose the activity.
Strength Training: Pull/Ab Workout

Activity	Frequency		Weight Lbs.	Intensity	Time (minutes between sets)
	Reps	Sets			
Regular-grip pulldown	10	3		3	1
One-arm dumbbell row	10	3		3	1
Reverse-grip pulldown	10	3		3	1
Regular dumbbell curl	10	3		3	1
Hammer curl	10	3		3	1
Concentration curl	10	3		3	1
Regular crunch	10	3		3	1
Reverse crunch	10	3		3	1
Elbow-to-knee crunch	10	3		3	1
Side crunch	10	3		3	1

Stretch: World's Fittest Man's Total Body Stretch

FITNESS TIP: Don't let a busy schedule get in the way of your workout. It's always easy to find an excuse not to work out. Try this: Pack your gym bag or take out your workout clothes the night before. Not only is it a great reminder and motivator, but if you're rushed in the morning all you have to do is grab that bag. No excuses!

Breakfast	*Breakfast Burrito Blitz* (page 105)
Snack #1	8 oz. low-fat yogurt 1 cup grapes
Lunch	*Tuna Salad Pita Pocket* (page 97) 1 apple 1 cup canned tomato soup
Snack #2	2 tbsp. peanut butter 6 whole-wheat crackers 1 tbsp. all-natural jam
Dinner	1 serving *World's Fittest Man Paella with Brown Rice* (page 268) *Apple Walnut Salad* (page 105)
Snack #3	½ banana

1,400 Version

Breakfast	Decrease Egg Beaters to ½ cup and salsa to ¼ cup
Snack #1	Omit yogurt
Lunch	Decrease tuna to 3 oz.; omit soup
Snack #2	Substitute 2 cups mixed vegetables with 1 tbsp. low-fat ranch dressing for entire snack
Dinner	substitute ½ cup steamed broccoli for salad; omit walnuts and raisins from salad

FOOD TIP: All salads are not created equal. Just because it's served on a bed of lettuce or in a bowlful of greens doesn't mean it's healthy. When you order a salad at a restaurant, make sure to check what's added. Lots of fresh vegetables like tomatoes, broccoli, carrots, and zucchini are generally better than croutons, cheese, meats, and eggs.

Think positively and masterfully, with confidence and faith, and life becomes more secure, more fraught with action, richer in achievement and experience.

—EDDIE RICKENBACKER

Joe's Wild Woodland Workout

Location: Wooded park or hiking trail (preferably with a hill)
Equipment:
Ordinary backpack
1 water bottle (for beginners bring a one-liter bottle, for intermediate a two-liter bottle, for advanced a one-gallon bottle)
For a real challenge you can load up your backpack with more bottles of water or other heavy items.
Time: 30–45 minutes

Warm-up. • 5-minute brisk walk or light jog.
Repeat the following workout 1–2 times for beginners, 3–6 times for intermediate/advanced:
Strength stop. • "Tree Push-up" (see "Incline Push-up" on page 215).
Do as many as you can until your muscles are fatigued. Keep the backpack on for more of a challenge.
Cardio. • 5-minute power walk or jog.
Strength Stop. • "Water Curl" (see "Curl" on page 229).
Using a water bottle, do as many as you can until your muscles are fatigued. Do one arm, then the other.
Cardio. • 5-minute power walk or jog. Go up a hill if you can find one.
Strength Stop. • "Stump Dip" (see "Chair Dip" on page 228).
Do as many as you can until your muscles are fatigued. If you can't find a tree stump, use a park bench for your dips.
Cardio. • 5-minute powerwalk or jog.

Strength Stop. • Walking Lunge (see "Dumbbell Lunge" on page 240).

Do as many as you can, alternating legs until your muscles are fatigued. Keep the backpack on for an added challenge, but don't use dumbbells.

Cool Down. • Easy walk for 5 minutes until your heart rate slows down. Then do the World's Fittest Man's Total Body Stretch.

FITNESS TIP: If you want to get the most out of your workouts, make sure you're well rested. To really "Shock Your Body" you also have to rest it. The Sunday "rest day" is part of it, but also make sure you get a good night's sleep of at least 6 to 8 hours. When you sleep, your body restores itself so you can work out harder and stronger the next time. If you're having problems getting to sleep, physical activity has been shown to help you achieve a better night's sleep. Make sure you don't work out right before going to sleep—that will have the opposite effect and probably keep you awake.

Day 27 • SATURDAY

Breakfast	*Super Waffle Combo* (page 108)
Snack #1	½ cup low-fat whipped cottage cheese 4 whole-wheat crackers
Lunch	*Chicken Salad Pita Pocket and Soup* (page 112)
Snack #2	*Ants on a Log* (page 112)
Dinner	1 serving *World's Fittest Man Super Stir-fry with Chicken* (page 261) 1 cup cooked brown rice
Snack #3	8 oz. low-fat yogurt ⅛ cup low-fat granola

1,400 Version

Breakfast	Omit syrup and skim milk
Snack #1	Omit crackers
Lunch	Decrease chicken to 3 oz.; omit soup
Snack #2	Decrease peanut butter to 1 tbsp., banana to ½, celery sticks to 4
Dinner	Substitute mixed green salad with 1 tbsp. reduced-fat ranch dressing for brown rice
Snack #3	Decrease yogurt to 4 oz. and granola to 1 tbsp.

FOOD TIP: Just as you should schedule an "appointment" to work out, you should do the same for food shopping. Schedule a time at the start of the week when you can load up on all your Fittest Foods. When you go to the supermarket, make sure you do it on a full stomach to avoid those impulse purchases like cake and cookies. Also, you'll find the outer edges of the supermarket usually have more of the nutritious food you'll need for your meals. Take a look next time you're at the supermarket and you'll see that many of the inner aisles are packed with junk food.

Optimism is the faith that leads to achievement. Nothing can be done without hope and confidence.

—HELEN KELLER

Sunday's Success Story

Your Success Story

Now it's time to hear about your success story. How did you do? Remember that fitness test you took at the start of my program? Guess what? You're going to take it again and see how you did. Compare it to the one you took four weeks ago. If you want, e-mail me your results. I would love to hear about your improvements.

Test	Date: _____
Flexibility	
Push-up	
Crunch	
Cardio Endurance	

Today's your reward day. Substitute your reward meal for one of the meals in the plan.

Breakfast	*Hi-NRG Smoothie* (page 112)
Snack #1	12 raw unsalted almonds ¼ cup raisins 8 oz. low-fat yogurt
Lunch	*Salad Niçoise* (page 108)
Snack #2	*World's Fittest Man Bean Dip and Pita* (page 108)
Dinner	1 serving *World's Fittest Man Lemon Grilled Salmon with Spicy Sweet Potato Sticks* (page 265) 1 cup steamed cauliflower or broccoli
Snack #3	2 tbsp. peanut butter 6 whole-wheat crackers 1 tbsp. all-natural jam

1,400 Version

Breakfast	Omit tofu
Snack #1	Omit yogurt
Lunch	Decrease tuna to 3 oz.; omit roll
Snack #2	Decrease black beans to ⅛ cup, salsa to ⅛ cup, corn to 1 tbsp., sour cream to 2 tbsp., and pita to ½
Snack #3	Decrease peanut butter to 1 tbsp.

FOOD TIP: All those sugared drinks, like soft drinks and fruit-flavored drinks, don't just add extra calories and inches to your waist; research shows that the more sugared drinks you have, the less likely your chances of getting the proper amounts of certain vitamins and minerals. If you're thirsty, go for water, and if you're craving sweets, go for a fresh piece of fruit.

FIT, FITTER, FITTEST
MAINTAINING THE WORLD'S FITTEST YOU

Y ou've finished your first challenge, completing my four-week "Shock Your Body" program. Now you're ready for the next challenge. The first step, getting started, is definitely the hardest. Making any kind of change in your life is always difficult. But now you're well on your way to becoming "the World's Fittest You."

This chapter of the book is important. Here I'll show you how to take what you've learned in the four-week program and apply it to the rest of your life. Read this chapter carefully, because you'll probably be referring to it for years and years to come.

My maintenance program is divided into three levels: Fit, Fitter, and Fittest. I encourage you to keep pushing yourself, but it's really fine if you want to stay at the Fit level. There's nothing wrong with that. You'll be maintaining a great level of fitness that you've achieved after the first four weeks of the program. But many of you will want to take what you've achieved to the next level. If you're ready for that challenge, and you want to become Fitter, then you'll move to the next level. Again, you'll have the choice of staying at this level or moving on again to become the Fittest you can be. If you decide to take on this challenge, you're going to really have to work hard. Not that you haven't been working so far, but this level will give your body a really tough challenge.

At each level you're going to continue using the FIT Equation: changing up the Frequency, Time, and Intensity so that you continue to "Shock Your Body." You're going to be increasing your overall intensity and endurance with each level. You'll also continue to follow my "Power of Positive Eating" program. But now, you'll have some options.

The first level—Fit—lasts for four weeks. You can stay there for as long as you want, or if you're ready for another challenge, you can go on to the Fitter level. The Fitter level is another four weeks. Again, you can stay there or move on to the Fittest level.

THE "POWER OF POSITIVE EATING" MAINTENANCE PROGRAM

This is easy. You've seen how to make small changes and substitutions in your eating habits to become a "Power Positive Eater." You've seen how eating six times a day—three snacks and three small meals—really helps to keep you feeling full all day long without giving in to fattening temptations. To continue following my eating program you now have the option of changing the days around. For instance, you can choose day fifteen, if you like, and have that meal plan any day of the week.

If you want even more flexibility, you can mix and match the meals and snacks to create your own meal plans. I've given you lots of different menu ideas and suggestions for you to choose from. Refer back to the World's Fittest You Food Guide on page 69 to help you make sure you're getting the proper amount of each food type. Use those ten steps in my "Power of Positive Eating" program to guide your food choices each and every day. For instance, pay special attention to Step 8, "Take Control," when you're eating out. Finally, try to include as many foods from my ten World's Fittest Foods in your meal choices. Remember, this is not a diet but a way of life.

A note about the "Weight Loss Option." If, after finishing the four-week program, you feel like you want to lose some more weight, then simply continue following the "Weight Loss Option." You can rearrange the days in any order you like, but you must follow all the meals for that specific day. If you ever get off track later on, then go back to the daily meal plans. Whether it's the "Weight Loss Option" or "Weight Control," following the day-by-day meal plans will give you more structure and help you get back on track to achieving the results you want.

THE CARDIO MAINTENANCE PROGRAM

As I've said, my program is all about variety and changing things up. Not only will this continuously "shock" your body into better physical shape with each new routine, but you'll keep yourself from getting bored with your workouts.

To keep things interesting I've designed fifteen different cardio workouts for you, some longer, some shorter—some higher intensity, some lower. You'll find these starting on page 172. It doesn't matter which cardio activity you choose, whether it's rowing or running, you're going to apply the FIT Equation to your workout. Like you did in those first four weeks, you'll start each cardio workout with a short warm-up at a low intensity. Then, you'll go into the main part of the workout, varying the intensity of each time interval. You'll end the workout with a short warm-down at a low intensity. The warm-down is not part of the actual workout chart I've given you. You'll just have to remember to do this yourself at the end of each cardio workout. It only takes three to five minutes at a low intensity to get your heart rate down, but always do this before you stop.

Here's how it works. Take a look at Day 2 of Week 1 of the FIT Level on page 179. You see that the Frequency is 2 (F = 2), so that means you'll do two days of cardio that week. Even though the "Outside the Box" workout includes cardio, I didn't include it in the equation, just to keep things simple. The Time is twenty minutes (T = 20), and the Intensity is easy (I = easy). What that means is you'll choose the "20-Minute Easy" workout on page 172. I encourage you to make photocopies of the cardio workouts. That way you can bring them with you to your workout—whether it's outside or inside. And, that way, you'll know exactly what to do.

USING MY FIT STRENGTH MAINTENANCE PROGRAM

By now you're accustomed to my Push, Pull, Leg, and Ab routines. As you progress through the Fit, Fitter, and Fittest levels you'll be increasing your muscle strength and tone by adding more weight, if you want. You'll also continue to mix up those FIT Equation variables like Frequency and Intensity and Time so your muscles don't get used to the same routine over and over again.

Here's how it works. Take a look at Day 1 of Week 1 of the FIT Level on page 179. You can see that Day 1 is a "Push/Ab" day, so you'll work your chest, shoulder, and triceps muscles as well as your abs—completing the strength activities on the list. For Day 1 you also see that the Frequency is 10/3 (F = 10/3) meaning "ten sets" with "three reps." The Intensity is 2 (I = 2), so you'll definitely feel something, but not an all-out effort. And the Time is 1 (T = 1), meaning you'll rest one minute after each rep. I've included blank Strength-Training Workout charts starting on page 183 for you to take with you to your workouts, so you can keep track of your progress. There's a separate chart for each muscle group combination; all you have to do is fill in the FIT Equation numbers for that specific day. Remember to do a short cardio warm-up (five to seven minutes is enough) before each and every strength-training workout. You always want to be sure your muscles are nice and warm before you start lifting weights.

TOTAL BODY STRETCH

You know how I feel about stretching. It's a must-do after every workout. You should continue to follow the same stretching routine as you did in the four-week program—those thirteen stretching activities. As you increase the intensity and time of your workouts—no matter which level you choose—it's more important than ever to stretch those muscles after your workout. This is a great way to help stay injury free. Believe me, you'll thank me later for all of my insistence on your stretching.

"OUTSIDE THE BOX" WORKOUTS

Remember those crazy Saturday workouts? The ones in a playground and at a baseball diamond? The ones that got you out of the gym and working cardio and strength at the same time? The ones I said would "Shock Your Body" in a whole new way? Well, I want you to continue to include these workouts as part of your weekly routine.

Now, it's up to you which one you decide to choose each week. It's always best to change things up, so feel free even to create your own "Outside the Box" workouts by simply combining your favorite activities from these four different workouts. Just make sure you follow the same format: alternating short cardio with calisthenics and simple strength-training activities. And remember that for the strength-training you perform the activity "Till Muscle Fatigue." (See page 47 for a quick review.) If one of my workouts gets too easy, simply add another round of the "circuit"—but don't go over sixty minutes.

I always want to hear from you. If you create your own "Outside the Box" workout that you'd like to share with other "World's Fittest You" folks, e-mail it to me. I'll try to post it on my Web site for everyone to see and try for themselves.

A LIFETIME OF FITNESS

These maintenance plans are really just road maps to help you keep on track. With all the tools and options I've given you, at some point you can certainly create your own workout plan—and I encourage you to do this if you suddenly get bored with your workouts. But one of the best antidotes for "Exercise Boredom" is to try a fitness challenge. Read on to the next chapter and I'll tell you about some great races and events to challenge yourself with and keep motivated.

20-MINUTE WORKOUTS

20-Minute Easy

T = 20

I = Easy

Frequency	Intensity	Time
2–3 times per week	2	minutes 1–5
	4	minutes 6–15
	2	minutes 16–20

20-Minute Medium

T = 20

I = Medium

Frequency	Intensity	Time
2–3 times per week	3	minutes 1–5
	6	minutes 6–15
	3	minutes 16–20

20-Minute Hard

T = 20

I = Hard

Frequency	Intensity	Time
2–3 times per week	4	minutes 1–5
	8	minutes 6–15
	4	minutes 16–20

30-MINUTE WORKOUTS

30-Minute Easy

T = 30

I = Easy

Frequency	Intensity	Time
2–3 times per week	2	minutes 1–5
	4	minutes 6–9
	6	minutes 10–13
	2	minutes 14–17
	4	minutes 18–21
	6	minutes 22–25
	2	minutes 26–30

30-Minute Medium

T = 30

I = Medium

Frequency	Intensity	Time
2–3 times per week	3	minutes 1–5
	5	minutes 6–9
	7	minutes 10–13
	3	minutes 14–17
	5	minutes 18–21
	7	minutes 22–25
	3	minutes 26–30

30-Minute Hard

T = 30

I = Hard

Frequency	Intensity	Time
2–3 times per week	4	minutes 1–5
	7	minutes 6–9
	9	minutes 10–13
	4	minutes 14–17
	7	minutes 18–21
	9	minutes 22–25
	4	minutes 26–30

40-MINUTE WORKOUTS

40-Minute Easy

T = 40

I = Easy

Frequency	Intensity	Time
2–3 times per week	2	minutes 1–8
	4	minutes 9–16
	2	minutes 17–24
	6	minutes 25–32
	2	minutes 33–40

40-Minute Medium

T = 40

I = Medium

Frequency	Intensity	Time
2–3 times per week	3	minutes 1–8
	5	minutes 9–16
	3	minutes 17–24
	7	minutes 25–32
	3	minutes 33–40

40-Minute Hard

T = 40

I = Hard

Frequency	Intensity	Time
2–3 times per week	4	minutes 1–8
	6	minutes 9–16
	4	minutes 17–24
	8	minutes 25–32
	4	minutes 33–40

50-MINUTE WORKOUTS

50-Minute Easy

T = 50

I = Easy

Frequency	Intensity	Time
2–3 times per week	2	minutes 1–10
	3	minutes 11–20
	4	minutes 21–25
	5	minutes 26–30
	3	minutes 31–40
	2	minutes 41–50

50-Minute Medium

T = 50

I = Medium

Frequency	Intensity	Time
2–3 times per week	3	minutes 1–10
	4	minutes 11–20
	5	minutes 21–25
	6	minutes 26–30
	4	minutes 31–40
	3	minutes 41–50

50-Minute Hard Workout

T = 50

I = Hard

Frequency	Intensity	Time
2–3 times per week	4	minutes 1–10
	5	minutes 11–20
	6	minutes 21–25
	7	minutes 26–30
	5	minutes 31–40
	4	minutes 41–50

60-MINUTE WORKOUTS

60-Minute Easy

T = 60

I = Easy

Frequency	Intensity	Time
2–3 times per week	2	minutes 1–10
	4	minutes 11–18
	6	minutes 19–26
	2	minutes 27–34
	4	minutes 35–42
	6	minutes 43–50
	2	minutes 51–60

60-Minute Medium

T = 60

I = Medium

Frequency	Intensity	Time
2–3 times per week	3	minutes 1–10
	5	minutes 11–18
	7	minutes 19–26
	3	minutes 27–34
	5	minutes 35–42
	7	minutes 43–50
	3	minutes 51–60

60-Minute Hard

T = 60

I = Hard

Frequency	Intensity	Time
2–3 times per week	4	minutes 1–10
	7	minutes 11–18
	9	minutes 19–26
	4	minutes 27–34
	7	minutes 35–42
	9	minutes 43–50
	4	minutes 51–60

FIT LEVEL (4 WEEKS–LIFETIME)

Week 1

Day 1	Day 2	Day 3	Day 4	Day 5	Day 6	Day 7
Push/Ab	Cardio	Pull/Leg	Cardio	Push/Ab	Outside the Box	REST
F = 10/3	F = 2	F = 10/3	F = 2	F = 10/3		
I = 2	I = easy	I = 2	I = medium	I = 2		
T = 1	T = 20	T = 1	T = 30	T = 1		

Week 2

Day 1	Day 2	Day 3	Day 4	Day 5	Day 6	Day 7
Cardio	Pull/Leg	Cardio	Push/Ab	Cardio	Outside the Box	REST
F = 3	F = 12/2	F = 3	F = 12/2	F = 3		
I = easy	I = 3	I = medium	I = 3	I = easy		
T = 30	T = 2	T = 20	T = 2	T = 40		

Week 3

Day 1	Day 2	Day 3	Day 4	Day 5	Day 6	Day 7
Pull/Leg	Cardio	Push/Ab	Cardio	Pull/Leg	Outside the Box	REST
F = 10/3	F = 2	F = 10/3	F = 2	F = 10/3		
I = 3	I = medium	I = 3	I = easy	I = 3		
T = 1	T = 20	T = 2	T = 40	T = 1		

WEEK 4

Day 1	Day 2	Day 3	Day 4	Day 5	Day 6	Day 7
Cardio	Push/Leg	Cardio	Pull/Ab	Cardio	Outside the Box	REST
F = 3 I = medium T = 30	F = 12/2 I = 4 T = 2	F = 3 I = hard T = 20	F = 12/2 I = 4 T = 2	F = 3 I = easy T = 40		

FITTER LEVEL (4 WEEKS–LIFETIME)

WEEK 1

Day 1	Day 2	Day 3	Day 4	Day 5	Day 6	Day 7
Push/Ab	Cardio	Pull/Leg	Cardio	Push/Ab	Outside the Box	REST
F = 10/3 I = 3 T = 1	F = 2 I = easy T = 30	F = 10/3 I = 3 T = 1	F = 2 I = medium T = 40	F = 12/2 I = 3 T = 2		

WEEK 2

Day 1	Day 2	Day 3	Day 4	Day 5	Day 6	Day 7
Cardio	Pull/Leg	Cardio	Push/Ab	Cardio	Outside the Box	REST
F = 3 I = medium T = 30	F = 12/2 I = 4 T = 2	F = 3 I = easy T = 40	F = 10/3 I = 4 T = 1	F = 3 I = medium T = 50		

Week 3

Day 1	Day 2	Day 3	Day 4	Day 5	Day 6	Day 7
Pull/Leg	Cardio	Push/Ab	Cardio	Pull/Leg	Outside the Box	REST
F = 10/3	F = 2	F = 12/2	F = 2	F = 12/2		
I = 3	I = hard	I = 3	I = easy	I = 3		
T = 1	T = 20	T = 2	T = 50	T = 2		

Week 4

Day 1	Day 2	Day 3	Day 4	Day 5	Day 6	Day 7
Cardio	Push/Ab	Cardio	Pull/Ab	Cardio	Outside the Box	REST
F = 3	F = 12/2	F = 3	F = 12/2	F = 3		
I = hard	I = 4	I = hard	I = 4	I = easy		
T = 30	T = 2	T = 40	T = 2	T = 50		

FITTEST LEVEL (4 WEEKS–LIFETIME)

Week 1

Day 1	Day 2	Day 3	Day 4	Day 5	Day 6	Day 7
Cardio	Push/Ab	Cardio	Pull/Leg	Cardio	Outside the Box	REST
F = 3	F = 10/3	F = 3	F = 10/3	F = 3		
I = easy	I = 4	I = medium	I = 4	I = hard		
T = 40	T = 3	T = 50	T = 3	T = 30		

WEEK 2

Day 1	Day 2	Day 3	Day 4	Day 5	Day 6	Day 7
Push/Ab	Cardio	Pull/Leg	Cardio	Push/Ab	Outside the Box	REST
F = 12/2 I = 5 T = 2	F = 2 I = medium T = 50	F = 12/2 I = 5 T = 2	F = 2 I = hard T = 40	F = 10/3 I = 3 T = 1		

WEEK 3

Day 1	Day 2	Day 3	Day 4	Day 5	Day 6	Day 7
Cardio	Pull/Leg	Cardio	Push/Ab	Cardio	Outside the Box	REST
F = 3 I = hard T = 50	F = 10/3 I = 3 T = 3	F = 3 I = medium T = 60	F = 8/3 I = 5 T = 2	F = 3 I = hard T = 50		

WEEK 4

Day 1	Day 2	Day 3	Day 4	Day 5	Day 6	Day 7
Pull/Leg	Cardio	Push/Ab	Cardio	Pull/Leg	Outside the Box	REST
F = 8/3 I = 5 T = 2	F = 2 I = hard T = 60	F = 12/2 I = 4 T = 2	F = 2 I = easy T = 60	F = 12/2 I = 4 T = 2		

WORLD'S FITTEST YOU WORKOUT LOG

Strength Training: Push/Ab Workout

Date: _____

F = _____

I = _____

T = _____

Activity	Frequency		Weight Lbs.	Intensity	Time (minutes between sets)
	Reps	Sets			
Dumbbell bench press					
Standing shoulder press					
Incline dumbbell press					
Front raise					
Dumbbell flye					
Side raise					
Triceps pushdown					
Triceps kickback					
Parallel bar dip					
Regular crunch					
Reverse crunch					
Elbow-to-knee crunch					
Side crunch					

WORLD'S FITTEST YOU WORKOUT LOG

Strength Training: Pull/Leg Workout

Date: _____

F = _____

I = _____

T = _____

Activity	Frequency		Weight Lbs.	Intensity	Time (minutes between sets)
	Reps	Sets			
Dumbbell squat or leg press					
Regular-grip pulldown					
Straight-leg dumbbell deadlift					
One-arm dumbbell row					
Leg extension					
Reverse-grip pulldown					
Lying leg curl					
Regular dumbbell curl					
One-leg dumbbell calf raise					
Hammer curl					
Concentration curl					

WORLD'S FITTEST YOU WORKOUT LOG

Strength Training: Push/Leg Workout

Date: _____

F = _____

I = _____

T = _____

Activity	Frequency		Weight Lbs.	Intensity	Time (minutes between sets)
	Reps	Sets			
Dumbbell bench press					
Standing shoulder press					
Dumbbell squat or leg press					
Incline dumbbell press					
Leg extension					
Front raise					
Leg curl					
Dumbbell flye					
Side raise					
One-leg dumbbell calf raise					
Triceps pushdown					
Triceps kickback					
Parallel bar dip					

WORLD'S FITTEST YOU WORKOUT LOG

Strength Training: Pull/Ab Workout

Date: _____

F = _____

I = _____

T = _____

Activity	Frequency		Weight Lbs.	Intensity	Time (minutes between sets)
	Reps	Sets			
Regular-grip pulldown					
One-arm dumbbell row					
Reverse-grip pulldown					
Regular dumbbell curl					
Hammer curl					
Concentration curl					
Regular crunch					
Reverse crunch					
Elbow-to-knee crunch					
Side crunch					

CHALLENGE YOURSELF!

CHAPTER 10

INTRODUCTION

Now that you're on your way to living a happier, healthier, and fitter life, you're ready for the final part of my maintenance program. As I've said before, in order to keep your body and mind active, you have to keep challenging yourself. I do it all the time. After finishing the Grand Slam of Ultrarunning I told you about in my story, I needed a new challenge. Something to keep me focused and on track. That's why I took on the Guinness World Records challenge. Even now I continue to challenge myself with new races and fitness events. Don't get me wrong, it's great that you continue to work out and stay fit. But from my experience, having a challenge is a great way to stay motivated.

In this chapter I'll show you how to "Challenge Yourself!" by training for different types of fitness events. Some events will be more challenging than others, so you'll have to pick the one that's right for you. For each event I've provided a brief description and some Web-site resources so you can get more specific information about races and challenges in your area.

I've grouped the challenges into different levels: Fit, Fitter, and Fittest. There's also an Extreme level for those of you who are looking for the ultimate physical challenge. To see which level you're up for, take this Challenge Yourself! Readiness Test. Your answers to these questions will help assess your fitness level for the different challenges in this chapter. Ultimately, you are going to have to be your own judge of what you can and can't do. If you're not up for a challenge now, that's okay, you can and will be soon. Remember, you can do anything you set your mind to.

CHALLENGE YOURSELF! READINESS TEST

Can I walk or run 3–5 miles without stopping or feeling out of breath?	Yes	No
Can I bike 10–15 miles without stopping or feeling out of breath?	Yes	No
Can I walk or run 8–10 miles without stopping or feeling out of breath?	Yes	No
Can I bike 25–30 miles without stopping or feeling out of breath?	Yes	No
Can I run 10–15 miles without stopping or feeling out of breath?	Yes	No
Can I bike 60 miles without stopping or feeling out of breath?	Yes	No

Believe it or not, if you answered yes to one or two questions, you're probably ready for a "Fit"-level challenge. If you answered yes to three or four questions, then, what the heck, try a "Fitter"-level challenge. Now guess what, if you answered yes to five to six questions, go for it, you're up for a "Fittest"-level challenge. You can always go down a level. If you're not sure, try a lower-level challenge before moving to the next level. After you've successfully completed a few challenges at the "Fittest" level, then see if you can handle one of the "Extreme" challenges. These are some of the most difficult races around, so don't try them unless you're really up for the challenge.

FIT

Running Web Sites

Many of these Web sites include information about all the different running challenges you'll find in this chapter . . . from the 5K to the Ultramarathon:

www.coolrunning.com
www.runnersworld.com
www.run_down.com
www.runningnetwork.com
www.americanrunning.org
www.rrca.org

5K Family Fun Run

A 5K Fun Run is a good entry-level race. The distance is fairly short—in miles it's 3.1. Usually these events are "fun" because there's really not a lot of emphasis on competition and speed. It's more about getting some fresh air, chatting with friends, and even taking home one of those cool race T-shirts. I like to give all of my race T-shirts away to my mother and grandmother as souvenirs. Over time you'll be able to fill up an entire closet with these shirts if you hold on to them. After you've done this type of race a few times with just finishing as your goal, you'll probably want to focus more on speed and improving your time. But for now, just finishing is a huge accomplishment.

www.racefforthecure.com

MS Bike Tour

The MS Bike Tour attracts both casual cyclists and hard-core riders. There are several levels of the tour that you can ride in. You can go for the minimum requirement of thirty miles or push yourself to ride sixty miles, but only if you've done enough training. You'll see that the more seasoned rider will complete a hundred miles while competing in the tour. What I like about this event is that it doesn't matter how quickly you finish because every mile you ride and every dollar you raise makes a difference in the fight against multiple sclerosis. I enjoy competing in these tours because I know that I'm also raising money to make a difference in someone else's life. Even though a bike tour is not the most strenuous type of race, you must still prepare your muscles—and your rear—for a full day of biking.

www.nmss.org
www.ms150.org

AIDS Walk

The AIDS Walk is generally a 6.2-mile (10K) fund raiser walkathon that started in Los Angeles in 1985 and that now has an annual counterpart in almost every city across the country. The walk takes about two to three hours to finish. Over the past two decades this event has helped to raise millions of dollars. A portion of the money you raise goes directly to vital services that help people who are living with HIV and AIDS.

www.aidswalk.net

10K Run

If you are not ready for a half marathon or marathon, but feel the need to push yourself beyond the realm of the 5K, then the 10K is the perfect race for you. The 10K, about six miles, is a test of both speed and endurance, combining the best aspects of the 5K and other more strenuous competitions.

www.us10k.org

The Urban Challenge

One of the craziest challenges around is the Urban Challenge. It's a relative newcomer to the fitness scene—a sort of modern-day treasure hunt. The event is as much about street smarts as it is about fitness.

And it's much more demanding than meets the eye. It works like this. You and a partner race—run, walk, use public transportation—to find clues around your city. Following the clues takes you over a seven- to ten-mile course to twelve checkpoints. At each checkpoint you must take a photo with a digital camera as proof. The team that correctly finds all twelve checkpoints in the least amount of time wins. And the winning team gets a nice monetary prize.

www.urbanchallenge.com

FITTER

Three-Day Breast Cancer Walk

Over the past few years thousands of people have participated in one of the many fund-raising Avon Breast Cancer Walks that are held throughout the country. The walk takes place over three days and covers a distance of sixty miles total—that's twenty miles each day. The events are very well organized and many of the participants include breast cancer survivors and their relatives. Even though this charitable event is considered a walk, the length makes it a bit more strenuous. I suggest that you should be able to complete a six- to eight-mile walk or run without stopping before you begin your training. After three days on your feet crossing that finish line will feel terrific.

www.breastcancer3day.org

Half Century

A half century is a fifty-mile bike ride that is completed in one day. Before entering this event you should familiarize yourself with the basics of bicycle mechanics as well as being comfortable with riding around other cyclists. A successful ride depends not only on your training program, but on the quality of your equipment. Make sure you invest in padded cycling shorts and a good bicycle seat.

www.usacycling.org
www.bicycling.com
www.cyclery.com

Half Marathon

If you are planning to attack the marathon, but need more preparation, then the half marathon is the perfect stepping-stone. The 13.1-mile distance provides a challenge beyond the popular 10K while allowing for more flexibility than marathon preparation. You can actually run several half marathons during a single race season. If you can run about an eight- or nine-minute mile, then the entire race will take about two hours. If you decide to power walk, it will probably take a little over three hours.

Duathalon/Triathlon

If you like both running and biking, then why not do them together? A duathalon is an event that combines both sports into a single race. The most common duathalon is this: run two miles, bike ten miles, then run another two miles (although you can find many different configurations). If swimming is your sport, then you might want to consider a triathlon. You start off with a one-mile swim, then a twenty-five-mile bike ride, finishing up with a 10K (6.2-mile) run. It will probably take you about four hours to get to the finish line. You can also find "minitriathlons" with less overall mileage. Whether you try the duathalon or the triathlon, be prepared to wear comfortable gear through both or all activities.

www.usatriathlon.org
www.duathalon.com
www.trifind.com
www.insidetri.com

FITTEST

Marathon

In the 1970s and 1980s, the marathon, a 26.2-mile run, captured the spirit of a nation searching for the ultimate personal challenge. You must be able to complete a 10K or half marathon and have at least three months of general fitness training experience, including strength training, running, and cardiovascular conditioning. But even if you've run before, over time you can slowly build up your stamina and endurance. I've had many clients who told me they were not runners and lo and behold, a year later, they finished their first marathon. Remember how I told you about Susan's story earlier? Contact your local city marathon running club for a team training program in your area. That's really the best way to get started.

www.nyrrc.org/nyrrc/marathon
www.marathonandbeyond.com
www.aims-association.org

Sprint Adventure Races

One of the fastest-growing sports in the country is adventure racing. If you like the outdoors and working with a team, then these races are definitely for you. After my first adventure race I was completely hooked. A sprint adventure race usually lasts about three to six hours. With a team of two or three people you do activities such as trail running, mountain biking, kayaking, climbing, and orienteering. What's different about these races is that it's a real team sport—you must compete and finish the races together, as a team. The best way to get started is to join the United States Adventure Racing Association (US-ARA). Membership will get you a subscription to *Adventure World* magazine and information about all the different types of races. One of the most popular sprint adventure races is the Balance Bar Adventure Sprints that takes place in many major cities across the country. Depending on the location, you can generally expect ten to fifteen miles of mountain biking, five to eight miles of trail running, one to three miles kayaking, and then ten special tests.

www.usara.com
www.balancebaradventure.com/sprints
www.adventure360.com

Century Ride

If you love to bicycle, then try a century ride: one hundred miles of cycling in one day. I can't think of a better way to take in the sights and sounds of the countryside than on a bike. You'll have to prepare and train a lot for this amount of riding, but the exhilaration of completing a hundred miles is well worth it. There are many organized century rides, but you can also try it on your own. If you do, consider going with a friend. You may find that you both will be able to ride faster without more effort. Once you begin, you should establish your pace. Try to find a groove, settle in, and don't push yourself too hard at the beginning. And don't forget to make sure your bike seat is comfortable—you'll be on it for many hours.

www.usacycling.org
www.active.com/century_challenge

Powerlifting

If you're not up for an endurance challenge, why not try something that's just pure, brute strength: powerlifting. More and more men—and women, too—are participating in powerlifting events held each year throughout the country. To compete you must perform three lifts—the squat, the dead lift, and the bench press. All three test your ultimate strength. Believe it or not, these are the same strength-training movements you've been doing in my program (instead of using dumbbells, in the event you'll be using barbells). You're allowed three attempts at each lift and the best one is counted. I've done a few of these events and I had a great time. I've even done as well as some of the guys twice my size.

www.powerlifting.com

EXTREME!

Ironman

An extreme version of the triathlon is called the Ironman. If you're looking for an intense challenge, then this is it: a 2.4-mile swim, a 112-

mile bike ride, and a 26.2-mile run. The Ironman competition originated in Hawaii in 1978. Since then the event has become so popular that versions of it are held all over the world. Just to be clear, even though it's called the Ironman, women can participate, too—all you need is an "iron" will to finish. After you've done a few of these, you can move on to the double and triple Ironman races (that means two and three times as much mileage). For many of these races, you must qualify, having had experience in long-distance racing and having completed at least one marathon.

vnews.ironmanlive.com
www.trifind.com
www.oarevents.com

Ultramarathon

One of my favorite challenges is the ultramarathon. Any race that's longer than a marathon, 26.2 miles, qualifies as an ultramarathon. The most common is the 50-mile distance. If you can believe it, some ultramarathons take place on running tracks—running in circles for that distance can really get your head spinning. But what really makes these events "ultra" intense is when you compete while running through unusual terrain like mountains and deserts. Remember the Badwater 135 through Death Valley I told you I completed twice? There's another race that's just as crazy called the Marathon des Sables, often referred to as "the Toughest Footrace in the World." What makes it so tough is that you're trekking nearly 150 miles across the Sahara Desert. If you decide to try one of these races, make sure you have a few marathons under your belt.

www.americanultra.org
run100s.com
www.ultramarathonworld.com
www.badwaterultra.com
www.racingtheplanet.com

Long-Course/Expedition Adventure Races

If you enjoyed the sprint adventure races, then you might be ready for an even bigger challenge. The long-course and expedition adventure races involve even more skills like rappelling down a hundred-foot cliff, scuba diving, sailing, and horseback riding, just to name a few. Even though you compete with a team of two to five people, you'll still need a good level of endurance. Long-course adventure races usually last anywhere from twelve hours to two days. The next level, expedition adventure races, last from three to fifteen days. You may have heard of the Eco-Challenge Expedition Race. It's televised each year because it's so popular. Other races are less well known. Remember the Raid Gauloises race I told you about? What an "adventure" that was! It took my team eight days to finish. For many of these adventure races you need to qualify, but don't let that stop you from trying.

www.balancebar24hour.com
www.ecochallenge.com
www.raidgauloises.com
www.oarevents.com

Ultracycling

If riding a hundred miles isn't enough of a challenge for you, then what about ultracycling? That's riding distances of two hundred miles and up. These ultracycling events will really test the limits of what you think is humanly possible. One of the most extreme ultracycling events is the Race Across America: a three-thousand-mile nonstop ride from one coast to the other. If you're looking for something that will really "burn you up," try the Furnace Creek 508. It's fewer miles than the Race Across America—"only" five hundred—but the terrain through Death Valley and the Mojave Desert will certainly challenge your physical—and mental—stamina.

www.ultracycling.com
www.raceacrossamerica.org
www.the508.com

APPENDIX A: CARDIO ACTIVITIES

GYM ACTIVITIES (INDOOR)

Treadmill (Running or Walking)

I refer to the treadmill as the old faithful. Just about any gym or hotel across the country that you go to is bound to have one of these machines. Some of the new machines have lots of high-tech features, but they all do just about the same thing, give you a great running or walking workout. By adjusting the speed and the grade you can increase or decrease the intensity of your workout. I suggest putting the treadmill in the manual mode so you can focus on applying the FIT Equation throughout your workout. Remember, the intensity is one of the variables you'll be changing quite a bit in my program. Bear in mind, too, that running or walking on a treadmill is gentler on your body than running on asphalt. If you've had a rough day and don't want to think, try one of the preprogrammed workouts for a change.

Skill Level: Easy

Impact Level: High (Running)–Low (Walking)

Calories Burned (per 30 minutes): Running at 7 mph is 460; power walking at 4.5 mph is 220

- Keep your back flat and head in line with your spine.
- Use your arms—they help balance your legs.
- Keep your shoulders relaxed.
- Don't keep your hands clenched up in a tight fist.
- Make sure you have good shoes, socks, and the proper running gear.
- Don't hold on to the handrails.
- Increase the elevation and speed controls slowly, otherwise you may lose your balance.

Rowing Machine

So many people I train are so accustomed to the treadmill that they forget about the other options in the gym. The rowing machine is great because not only does it give you a cardiovascular workout, but it uses the muscles in your upper body, lower body, and abs too. If you're just starting out, you'll probably only want to go for a few minutes on this machine, since you'll be using muscles you might not be accustomed to. Before training for the Guinness World Records fitness competition, I had barely used this piece of equipment. In the beginning I was beat after just about fifteen minutes when I first started training. But slowly I worked my way up and eventually went for ten miles in sixty minutes. Be prepared, the faster and harder you pull, the greater you'll feel the resistance. Practice your form. The better your form, the more you'll enjoy this machine.

Skill Level: Medium

Impact Level: Low

Calories Burned (per 30 minutes): 208

ROWING TIPS:

- When you start, your legs should be bent into your knees and arms straight in front of you at shoulder level. To complete the rowing "stroke," straighten your legs, keeping your arms extended in front of you. When your arms reach your knees, lean back slightly, pulling your arms into your chest.
- Keep your grip on the handle relaxed or else your forearms will get sore.
- Try not to use your biceps. Concentrate on the larger muscles of your back and legs to get the job done.
- Don't lean back too far; it puts excess strain on your back.
- If you can, maintain proper technique by watching yourself in a mirror.
- You can vary the resistance by adjusting the resistance lever on the side of the flywheel. A resistance of 1 is like you're rowing a speedy kayak and a resistance of 10 is like pulling a tugboat.

Elliptical Trainer

If you want a great workout with little impact on your joints or bones, then you should try this piece of equipment. The elliptical trainer combines running, cross-country skiing, riding a bike, and climbing stairs in an oval-like motion. It builds endurance and leg power and is easy on your joints. When I want to take a break from my long training runs, I use this machine. There's even a model that has arm bars so that you can work your upper body too. One trick that I've just discovered is that you can go in reverse, to give your muscles a different workout. The backward motion really develops your glutes or buttock muscles and your hamstrings. It's a real butt blaster, especially if you increase the incline.

Skill Level: Easy

Impact Level: Low

Calories Burned (per 30 minutes): 324

- Stand tall and keep your head up.
- Try not to grip the handrails.
- Adjust the cross ramp to target different leg muscles.
- Adjust the resistance to vary the intensity.

Stair Climber

A stair climber is great for working your hamstrings, buttocks, and calf muscles in addition to getting a good cardiovascular workout. Like the elliptical trainer the stair climber is a great alternative to high-impact activities like running or even climbing real stairs. One thing you have to be careful about is proper form. I see many people bent over and putting all their weight on the handrails. Be careful, this is bad form and can actually do more damage than any good you might get from the workout. Instead, when you're using this machine, stand up straight and lightly hold on to the handrails, for balance only, not support. Be sure to adjust the speed so you can keep up.

Skill Level: Easy

Impact Level: Low

Calories Burned (per 30 minutes): 211

STAIR CLIMBER TIPS:
- Stand up straight, lean slightly forward at the hips.
- Place your entire foot on pedal.
- Take full, even steps, not short choppy ones.
- Really concentrate on working your rear.

Indoor Cycling

One of my favorite indoor activities with little or no impact on the joints is the stationary bicycle. You can get a great workout on one of these bikes, whether it's the regular upright bike or the newer recumbent model. The recumbent bike is good if you have problems with your lower back. Whichever bike you choose, it's easy to change the intensity. Crank up the intensity and it feels like you're climbing a huge hill. Lower it and you're speeding back down. You can increase the intensity in the FIT Equation a few easy ways. You can increase the resistance, making it harder to pedal, like you're going uphill. You can also increase the speed with which you pedal, called RPM (revolutions per minute). The faster your RPM, the higher you'll feel the intensity. You might also want to try a spinning class at your local gym. The spinning bike is a little different and feels more like a bike you'd ride outside. You control the resistance with a knob. The group aspect of the class may help give you additional motivation.

Skill Level: Easy

Impact Level: Low

Calories Burned (per 30 minutes): 205 at 12 mph

INDOOR CYCLING TIPS:

- Make sure the seat height is adjusted correctly. Your legs should be slightly bent when you peddle down. If your leg is completely straight, you're going to put a strain on your knee.
- Keep the ball of your foot firmly on the pedal or inside the toe clip.
- If the resistance is too high, it can cause you to strain your legs.
- Hold the handlebars loosely; don't grip too tightly.
- Try using the toe clip so you can push and pull the pedal at the same time. This gives you the most bang for your buck.

Cross-Country Ski Machine

What's terrific about the cross-country ski machine is that it gives your entire body a workout, while at the same time it has little or no impact on your joints. You'll feel it in your arms and legs, and if you're not used to the movement, you'll probably feel a little sore the next day. That's fine—it takes a little practice to get used to the skiing movement. Start by working your legs, then incorporating your arms. But don't let the awkwardness stop you. What I like about the machine is that it's good for a nice steady workout. There are different types of cross-country ski machines, but the most popular is the NordicTrack. The older versions have cable pulleys and the new models are more streamlined.

Skill Level: Medium

Impact Level: Low

Calories Burned (per 30 minutes): 282

CROSS-COUNTRY SKI MACHINE TIPS:
- Stand tall, leaning with your hips into the hip pads.
- Keep your head up and your face forward, don't look at your feet.
- Maintain an opposite arm-to-leg movement.
- Practice, practice, practice. This is a great workout once you get the technique down. It can be tough for uncoordinated people like me.

OUTDOOR ACTIVITIES

Power Walking

Believe it or not, walking is one of the most convenient activities to get started with your cardio program. You can walk virtually anywhere and it doesn't require lots of special equipment and clothing. It's very low impact on your body. On top of all that, research shows that walking really does benefit your health. One study showed that walking briskly for just six times a month cut the risk of premature death in men and women dramatically. Growing up on the farm, there was an old farmer down the road who walked every morning religiously. I think he lived to be about ninety and looked great until the end.

When you first start my program, if you're new to fitness, you'll start off with simple walking to build up your stamina such as walking around the block during your lunch break and taking the long way to your car or bus stop after work. After that you'll be on your way to one of my favorite cardio activities, power walking. This was one of the events in the Guinness World Records fitness challenge and it's really no more difficult than just plain walking. When you power walk you're just walking at a higher intensity, pumping your arms to help propel yourself faster.

Skill Level: Easy

Impact Level: Medium

Calories Burned (per 30 minutes): 220 at 4.5 mph

POWER WALKING TIPS:
- Take short, quick steps.
- Practice heel-to-toe roll.
- Squeeze your buttocks to help strengthen your lower back muscles.
- Pull your abdominal muscles up and in as you walk.
- Pump your arms with an opposite arm-to-leg movement.
- Keep your chest out, shoulders back, and head up.

Climbing Stairs

If you are short on time for the day's workout, take the stairs. Even if it's only a few flights, it's better than nothing. As I've said before, even short bursts of cardio activity, like climbing the stairs throughout your workday, can be combined to help you reach your goal. One study even found that men who climbed at least twenty floors per week had a 20 percent lower risk of having a stroke. If you want to really firm up your butt, nothing works like climbing stairs. This is one of my favorite workouts. Find a tall building and hit the stairs for a few repeats. You'll be surprised by the workout you get.

Skill Level: Easy

Impact Level: Medium

Calories Burned (per 30 minutes): 280

CLIMBING STAIRS TIPS:
- Pick up the pace on the way up and take it nice and slow on the way down.
- Climbing two steps at a time is good for building strong thigh and butt muscles.
- Try not to use the handrail.
- For added resistance, throw on a backpack.

Running

From reading my story you know that I love to run. For me, the longer the better, and the more extreme the more fun. Believe it or not, my favorite race was the Badwater Ultramarathon—135 miles through the California desert. I liked it so much I've now done it twice. I realize that these extreme running races may not be for you, but running is definitely a great way to burn off calories while at the same time getting your butt out of the gym. For me it's also a great stress reducer and my personal time to solve all the world's problems. As I'm running through the park and down my local streets, the tension of the day seems to just melt away. And it's so easy; all you need is a good pair of sneakers, a T-shirt, and shorts. Try to find a path that is soft on your feet, like an outdoor track or dirt road. The constant pounding on pavement can really take its toll on your feet and legs. Overall, running is great for your health. Research shows that running twenty to forty minutes a day three to five times per week may dramatically reduce your chances of dying from cancer .

Skill Level: Easy

Impact Level: High

Calories Burned (per 30 minutes): 330 at 5.5 mph; 460 at 7 mph; 640 at 10 mph

RUNNING TIPS

- Look ahead of you, not directly down. This helps promote better posture to prevent upper back and neck pain. Not only that, you'll be able to see where you're going and avoid running into something or getting run over.
- Wear reflective running gear if you're going to be running at night.
- Always run against traffic, that way oncoming cars can see you better on the road.
- Keep your shoulders relaxed.
- On humid and hot days make sure to drink plenty of water during your run.
- Get good shoes, socks, and proper running attire. It makes a big difference.

Swimming

If you know how to swim, then you're one step ahead of the game. Swimming is one of the best full-body cardio activities you can find. It works just about every muscle in your body with little or no impact. If you really want the calorie-burning and endurance benefits of swimming, though, you need to do more than "dog-paddle" or float on your back. Growing up, my mom taught me to swim in the creek near our house. The only problem was that there were lots of water moccasins, so I had to swim really fast to get away from them. I didn't swim in a pool until I was a teenager. If you don't know how to swim already, the local YMCA or parks and recreation center often offers classes. And if you're not a swimmer but still like the water, you might want to consider a water aerobics class.

Skill Level: Medium

Impact Level: Low

Calories Burned (per 30 minutes): 280 for light/moderate effort; 350 for fast/vigorous effort

SWIMMING TIPS:

- Breathe out through your mouth.
- Try adding handheld paddles to increase the intensity and resistance on your arms.
- Kick from the hips, not from the knee, and try not to break the surface of the water.
- Alternate strokes to break up some of the monotony of going back and forth.
- Find a local swim club or swim team to join; that will also keep you motivated.
- The crawl or freestyle stroke gives you the best workout with maximum cardio benefit.
- Use goggles to keep your eyes from getting irritated from the chlorine.

Kayaking

A kayak is a paddle boat like a canoe, only it's smaller and generally easier to handle. I only learned to kayak a few years ago when I was training for the Guinness World Record challenge. To be honest, I learned by watching a few expert kayakers in my area and joining my friend Ben for a few workouts. They made it look so easy, but boy, is it a tough workout. After my first go at kayaking my arms and shoulders really ached. But it's great fun and really builds your upper body in ways that lifting weights can't. Your arms, back, abs, and legs will feel it too. Depending on the strength of the current and your speed, you can really get your heart rate up. Most of all, when you're out on the water you'll feel an incredible sense of exhilaration. That feeling will last for days after your workout. For more information about kayaking you might want to visit the American Canoe Association Web site *(www.acanet.org)*.

Skill Level: High

Impact Level: Low

Calories Burned (per 30 minutes): 150

KAYAKING TIPS:
- Always wear a personal flotation device (a life vest) and helmet.
- Check the currents and plan a suitable route.
- Always kayak with a friend.
- Take a class at a local YMCA or certified instructor to learn basic kayaking skills.
- Try both ocean and white-water kayaking once you learn the basics.

Hiking

If you want to get out of the gym, I can't think of a better activity than hiking. Hiking is perfect for all levels of fitness. Not only is it a good workout for your legs (especially if there are hills) and your heart, but you'll get to enjoy the beautiful clean, fresh air of the outdoors. You won't even think it's a workout at all. It might not burn as many calories as forty-five minutes on the treadmill, but you'll be having a great time, and that's what fitness is all about. You can stop to smell the flowers and enjoy beautiful vistas, but remember, you'll have to keep your intensity up to get a good cardio workout. Grab a friend, your backpack, and hiking boots and head for the trails and hills.

Skill Level: Easy

Impact Level: Medium

Calories Burned (per 30 minutes): 180

HIKING TIPS:
- Wear supportive shoes with a closed toe. Avoid wearing sandals or flip-flops.
- Check the weather forecast before you leave.
- Wear appropriate clothing. If it's cold, dress in layers so that when your body starts to heat up you can remove a layer of clothing and tie it around your waist.
- Bring water, a map of the area, compass, and a simple first-aid kit with you.
- Carry a backpack for water and food (the extra weight will help burn even more calories).
- Know your limits; don't head for Mount Everest on your first outing.

In-line Skating

Once you get the hang of in-line skating (and I suggest lessons if you've never done it before), you can get a workout just as intense as running. One study reported that in-line skating can provide the same level of cardio activity as running. And because you're pushing your legs to the side, you'll be toning your hip and buttock muscles. I learned to skate near the beach in San Diego. The hardest part was learning how to stop. After a few falls—yes, even the World's Fittest Man falls—I really came to enjoy the sport. For this activity you're going to need a pair of good in-line skates, and make sure they're ones that fit properly. Don't just borrow a pair from a friend unless you're exactly the same size. Most injuries and sore feet are caused by improperly fitting skates. Before getting started with in-line skating, check out the International Inline Skating Association Web site *(www.iisa.org)*. There, you can find great information about safety and even the best places to skate in your local area.

Skill Level: Hard

Impact Level: Low

Calories Burned (per 30 minutes): 300

IN-LINE SKATING TIPS:
- Always wear a helmet, wrist guards, elbow pads, and knee pads.
- Use bike paths and parks to avoid cars and traffic.
- If you're skating in the street, obey all traffic laws, including stopping at intersections.
- Hills are difficult unless you've really mastered how to stop.
- Don't skate with your dog's leash or with anything else in your hand.

Bicycling

Bicycling is another one of my favorite outdoor activities. You can really build up your calves, hamstrings, and quads with very little impact on your body. Once you get your equipment, including a helmet and comfortable shoes, you're on your way. If you are strapped for time—on days you can't seem to fit in a workout—you might want to consider taking your bicycle to work or the supermarket. Bicycling is also a perfect activity to do with your kids. There are many different types of bikes today. The three most popular are road, mountain, and hybrid bikes. A road bike is lightweight and designed primarily for hard surfaces. If you're more adventurous, a mountain bike is built for riding on trails and dirt roads. Not sure, most people choose a hybrid bike, which is a cross between a mountain and road bike.

Skill Level: Medium

Impact Level: Low

Calories Burned (per 30 minutes): 120 at 6 mph; 205 at 12 mph

BICYCLING TIPS:

- Always ride with a helmet—you can get a good one for around $35.
- Buy a pair of padded cycling shorts—it will make your ride much more comfortable.
- Learn how to fix a flat; you never know when you'll have a blowout.
- Concentrate on your surroundings, and don't let your eyes wander from the road or trail.
- Don't squeeze the brakes, particularly the front brake, with too much pressure. Instead pump both brakes with a moderate amount of force. This way you don't go flying over the handlebars.
- Ride relaxed, with as little tension in your upper body and arms as possible.
- Plan a route that's varied, involving hills and flats.
- Keep your pedal stroke smooth.

Jumping Rope

We all remember jumping rope as a kid, and, believe it or not, it's actually a perfect at-home cardio activity. You can buy a basic jump rope for around $5 or $6. Some are more expensive and have fancy leather handles. These are fine, too, but I like to stick to the basics. A jump rope is great for travel or if you have minimal space at home. Most people think you have to be incredibly coordinated to jump rope. Not so. I've trained many people who told me they were klutzes and would never be able to master the technique. It's really easy. First try going back and forth between brief periods of jumping with resting moves, such as turning the rope alongside your body without jumping. As you progress, do fewer resting moves and more jumping. Surprisingly, after a little practice, you'll be jumping for fifteen minutes straight. Watch out, Mike Tyson!

Skill Level: Medium

Impact Level: High

Calories Burned (per 30 minutes): 375

JUMPING ROPE TIPS:

- Adjust your rope to get the right length. When you step in the center of the rope, the handles should just reach your armpits.
- Wear a good pair of cross-training shoes. Never jump with bare feet.
- Rubber tiles or carpeting has a softer impact on your feet than concrete or wood floors.
- Keep your shoulders relaxed and elbows in, close to your body.
- Control your jumps and don't go too high.
- Turn the rope with your wrists, not your arms.
- Alternate between the balls of your feet and heels to avoid strain.
- Grab the kids and try a little double Dutch.

APPENDIX B: STRENGTH-TRAINING ACTIVITIES

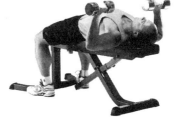

CHEST

Dumbbell Bench Press
(Gym/Home Version)

Starting Position. • Lie on the bench with your knees bent, your feet flat on the floor, and your back flat. Grip the dumbbells with your palms facing forward, positioning the dumbbells just above your shoulders with your arms bent.

The Movement. • Press the dumbbells directly straight above your shoulders for two counts, completely extending your arms. Pause, then slowly lower the dumbbells for four counts back to the armpit area, the starting position.

TRAINING TIPS:
- Make sure to keep the dumbbells over your chest area—it's easy for them to sway back toward your head or toward your belly.
- To get the maximum chest stretch, lower the dumbbells as far as you can.
- Make sure not to arch your back or bring your feet off the floor.
- Don't bounce the dumbbells off your chest.
- Keep your butt on the bench throughout the movement.

Incline Dumbbell Press

(Gym/Home Version)

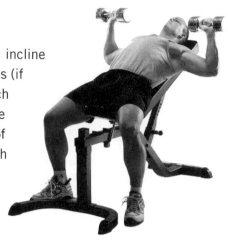

Starting Position. • Angle the incline on your bench to 30–60 degrees (if you don't have an incline bench at home, place a few phone books underneath one side of the bench). Lie flat on the bench with your knees bent and feet flat on the floor. Grip the dumbbells with your palms facing forward, positioning the dumbbells at shoulder level with your arms bent.

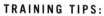

The Movement. • Press the dumbbells directly above your upper chest for two counts, completely extending your arms. Pause, then slowly lower the dumbbells for four counts back to your shoulders, the starting position.

TRAINING TIPS:

- Make sure to press the dumbbells straight up, not over the back of your head.
- Keep your head on the bench; don't let it lift up.
- Squeeze your chest when your arms are extended to keep your muscles working.

Dumbbell Flye

(Home/Gym Version)

Starting Position. • Lie flat on your back with your feet firmly on the floor. Hold the dumbbells so that your palms are facing in. Your arms should be slightly bent at shoulder level. You should feel a strong stretching sensation across your chest.

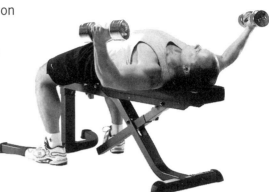

The Movement. • Raise the dumbbells up and together for two counts like you're giving someone a hug. Pause, then slowly lower the dumbbells for four counts back to the starting position.

TRAINING TIPS:

- You should feel the stretch in your chest without any pain in your shoulders.
- Keep a slight bend in your elbows.
- This is one of the best chest activities. It really isolates the chest muscles. For you guys, this movement will help give you a nice cut down the middle your chest.

Push-up

(Gym/Home Version)

Starting Position. • Place your hands shoulder-width apart, balancing your entire body on your toes and palms of your hands. Your body should be in a straight line without your butt sticking up in the air.

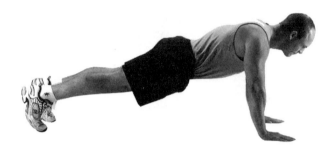

The Movement. • Slowly bend your arms, lowering your body for two counts until you're about an inch or two off the floor. Pause, then slowly straighten your arms for two counts, returning to the starting position.

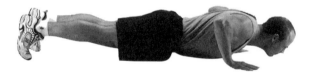

TRAINING TIPS:

- This is a great strength activity if you're on the road or at the office and can't get to the gym.
- Slow and steady wins the race . . . no need to hurry through your push-ups. Go slowly, keeping constant tension in your upper-body muscles.
- For a real challenge, add a clap when you're returning to the starting position.

Fittest Variations:

Modified Push-up

If you're having trouble doing the full number of repetitions, try this modified variation. Bend your knees and position your heels toward your butt. Make sure to keep your weight on the front of your knees, not directly on the kneecap.

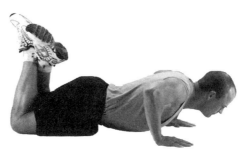

Incline Push-up

Place your hands on the top of a bench, chair, or couch (make sure whatever you choose is sturdy enough to hold your weight). Your body should be at about a 45-degree angle with the floor so you feel the push-up more in your lower chest. Like the modified variation, this one is easier than the regular push-up because you don't have to support your entire body weight.

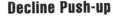

Decline Push-up

For a real challenge, rest your feet on a bench or chair, no more than two feet off the ground. You'll feel it more in your shoulders and the top of your chest, since you're working harder against gravity.

SHOULDERS

Standing Shoulder Press
(Gym/Home Version)

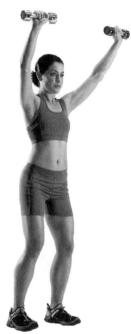

Starting Position. •
Stand with your feet
about shoulder-width apart,
knees slightly bent,
chest out, and head up.
Grip the dumbbells so
that your palms are facing
forward and are level
with your shoulders.

The Movement. •
Press the dumbbells
over your head for two counts,
until they almost touch. Keep your arms
straight but don't lock your elbows.
Pause, then slowly lower your arms for four
counts, back to the starting position.

TRAINING TIPS:
- Keep your back straight and your abdominal muscles tight so that you take the pressure off your lower back.
- When you lower your arms back to the starting position, make sure the dumbbells are almost touching your shoulders—if you don't go all the way down, you're not getting the full movement.

Fittest Variation.

If you like, you can perform the same activity sitting in a chair or on a bench. You can also alternate lifting one arm over your head, returning it to the starting position, then lifting the other arm. However, you actually get the best results by doing this activity standing. When you're standing you use more muscles—your abs and legs—to help stabilize your body.

Front Raise

(Gym/Home Version)

Starting Position. • Stand with your feet about shoulder-width apart, knees slightly bent, chest out, and head up. Grip the dumbbells straight by your side, palms facing inward.

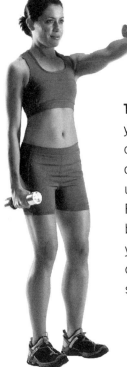

The Movement. • Raise your left arm, rotating the dumbbell directly in front of you for two counts until it's eye level. Pause, then lower it for four counts, back to the starting position. Complete your repetitions, then repeat with the opposite arm. When you finish both sides, that's one set.

TRAINING TIPS:
- Keep your body still and don't sway back and forth.
- Well-developed shoulders can help make your waist look smaller.

Side Raise

(Gym/Home Version)

Starting Position. • Stand with your feet about shoulder-width apart, knees slightly bent, chest out, and head up. Grip the dumbbells so that your arms are directly at your side, palms facing inward.

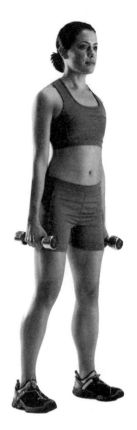

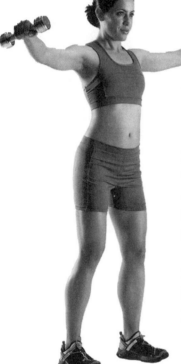

The Movement. • With a slight bend in your elbow, raise your arms for two counts until they are level with your shoulders and parallel to the floor. Pause, then slowly lower for four counts, back to the starting position.

TRAINING TIPS:

- Keep your body still. Try not to rock back and forth as you perform the movement. If you're using too much weight, you will probably start to rock and that takes the work off your shoulders.
- To help prevent your body from swaying and to stabilize your balance, you may want to have one leg slightly in front of the other.

BACK

Regular-Grip Pulldown

(Gym Version)

Starting Position. • Sit yourself at the lat pulldown machine. Adjust the seat so that your knees fit comfortably under the pads and your feet are flat on the floor. Grip the bar with your hands a little bit wider than shoulder-width apart and your palms facing away from you.

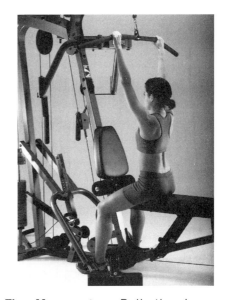

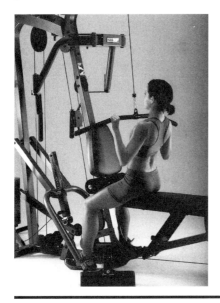

The Movement. • Pull the bar down for two counts toward your chest by bending your elbows. Your back should be slightly arched, with your head tilted back. Pause when the bar is a little below chin level, then, for four counts, slowly return to the starting position.

TRAINING TIPS:

- Keep your upper body as steady as possible—don't sway back and forth.
- Focus on pushing up your chest to meet the bar without leaning back. This position gives your back a better workout without involving your shoulders.
- Avoid bringing the bar behind your head to prevent injuring your neck.

Pull-up

(Home Version of Regular-Grip Pulldown)

Starting Position. • Securely attach a chin-up bar about five feet above the floor, depending on your height. Grip the bar with your hands just over shoulder-width apart and your palms facing forward. Hang from the bar with your arms fully extended.

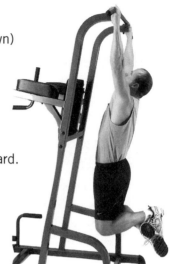

The Movement. • Pull yourself up until your chin is just above the bar. Pause, then slowly lower yourself for two counts back to the starting position.

TRAINING TIPS:

- Pull-ups are a great back-developing activity that you can do practically anywhere you can find a sturdy bar.
- Concentrate on using your back muscles and not just pulling yourself up with your arms.

Fittest Variations:

Place a chair or bench underneath the bar for support. With your feet behind you resting on the chair, use your feet to help push yourself up.

You can change things up by varying the width of your grip. For a real challenge, try gripping the bar as wide as you can. Then, try gripping the bar with your hands as close as possible.

Reverse-Grip Pulldown

(Gym Version)

Starting Position. • Sit yourself at the lat pulldown machine. Grip the bar with your
hands shoulder-width apart
and your palms facing
toward you (this is called an
underhand or reverse grip).

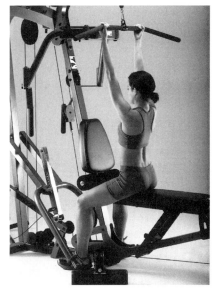

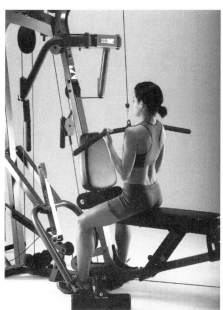

The Movement. • Pull the bar
down toward your chest for two
counts by bending your elbows. Your back should be
slightly arched with your head
tilted back. Pause when the
bar is at chin level, then
slowly, for four counts, return
to the starting position.

TRAINING TIPS:

- Keep your abs tight as you pull the bar down. This takes the pressure off your lower back.
- The reverse grip targets your biceps, too, so you get better results.

Reverse Chin-up

(Home Version of Reverse-Grip Pull-down)

Starting Position. • Securely attach your chin-up bar about five feet above the floor, depending on your height. Grip the bar with your hands shoulder-width apart and your palms facing inward and toward you. Hang from the bar with your arms fully extended.

The Movement. • Pull yourself up until your chin is just above the bar. Pause, then slowly lower yourself back to the starting position for two counts.

TRAINING TIPS:

- Don't swing back and forth through the movement.
- When you lower your body, make sure to extend your arms fully; don't shorten the movement.

Fittest Variation:

Attach the chin-up bar about three to four feet off the floor. Lie underneath the bar and grip the bar with your palms facing your feet about shoulder-width apart. Hang from the bar, keeping your arms straight and body fully extended so only your heels touch the floor. Pull yourself up toward the bar by bending your elbows. Pause, then slowly lower yourself to the starting position.

One-Arm Dumbbell Row

(Gym/Home Version)

Starting Position. • Grip a dumbbell in your right hand with your palm facing inward. Bend your body forward from the hips, placing your left hand on the front of the bench to stabilize your body. Your right foot should be on the floor about twelve inches from the bench, your left knee resting on the bench, and your back should be straight. Your right arm should now hang straight from your shoulder next to the bench.

The Movement. • Lift the dumbbell up toward your hip for two counts, keeping your elbow in and as far back as it will go. Pause, then slowly lower back for four counts to the starting position. Complete your repetitions, then repeat with your left arm, keeping your right arm and knee on the bench this time. When you finish both sides, that's one set.

TRAINING TIPS:

- Concentrate on using your back, not your arm, muscles.
- Keep your back as straight as possible. It helps to watch yourself in a mirror so that you maintain a flat back throughout the movement.
- A strong back will help you maintain good posture.

TRICEPS

Triceps Pushdown

(Gym Version)

Starting Position. • Attach a straight bar to the cable machine. Position yourself in front of the bar with your feet about shoulder-width apart and your knees slightly bent. Grip the bar with your palms facing down. Then, bring the bar down until your hands are level with your shoulders and elbows at your side.

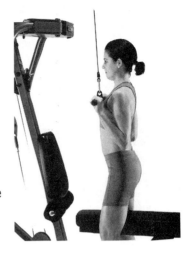

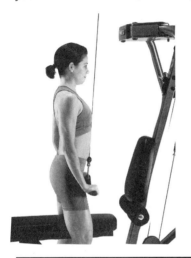

The Movement. • Extend your arms fully straight for two counts, keeping your elbows close to your body. Pause, then return slowly for four counts to the starting position.

TRAINING TIPS:

- Move only your forearms, keeping your upper arms straight. This will ensure that you work your triceps completely.
- For balance you can place one foot in front of the other.

Fittest Variations:

If you want, you can vary this activity by using an angled bar or a rope instead of a straight bar. With a rope, make sure your palms are facing inward. You can also use a reverse grip, palms facing upward, with the straight bar.

Overhead Triceps Extension

(Home Version of Triceps Pushdown)

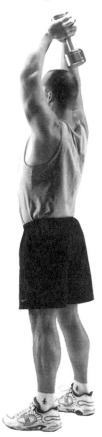

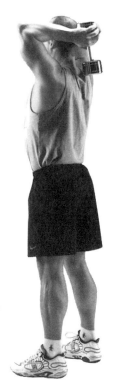

Starting Position. • Stand with your feet shoulder-width apart and with your back as straight as you can. Grip a dumbbell in both hands so that your palms are facing up and elbows bent 90 degrees.

The Movement. • Bending your arms from your elbows, raise the dumbbell slowly for two counts straight up over your head. Pause, then slowly lower back to the starting position for four counts, keeping your upper arms in a fixed position.

TRAINING TIPS:

- Focus on keeping the upper arm steady while bending only your elbows. This is difficult to do, especially if you're using too much weight. Try performing the movement without the dumbbell first. Look at yourself in the mirror and make sure you have the correct movement.
- Keep your neck relaxed and look forward. Turning your neck or crunching it during the movement will put extra strain on your neck muscles.

Triceps Kickback

(Home/Gym Version)

Starting Position. • Rest your right hand and knee on a bench with your back straight. Grip a dumbbell with your left hand. Bend your left elbow so that your upper arm is parallel to and your fore-arm perpendicular to the floor.

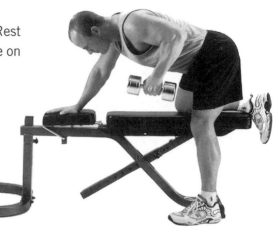

Movement. • Extend your left arm back for a count of two until your entire upper arm is completely straight and parallel to the floor. Lower your arm back to the starting position for a count of four. Complete your repetitions, then repeat with the other arm. When you finish both sides that's one set.

TRAINING TIPS:

- When you switch arms, make sure to change leg position too.
- Keep you elbow tight by your side throughout the entire movement.
- When your arm is fully extended you should feel a pump in your triceps.

Parallel-Bar Dip

(Gym Version)

Starting Position. • Grip the parallel bars with both your hands, palms facing inward. Suspend yourself between the bars with your elbows slightly bent. Your knees should also be slightly bent, your chin tucked in near your chest. Keep your body as straight as possible.

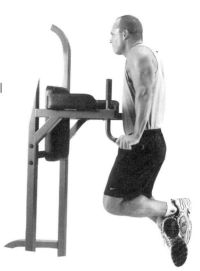

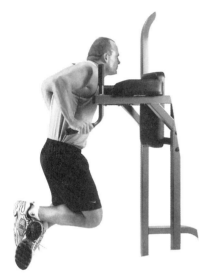

The Movement. • Bending at your elbows, slowly lower yourself between the bars for four counts until your arms are just about parallel to the ground. Your elbows should be bent at 90 degrees. Pause, then push yourself up for two counts without fully straightening your arms.

TRAINING TIPS:

- You can work your chest muscles more by leaning forward 45 degrees rather than keeping your body straight.
- Try not to go too fast or swing back and forth. Focus on good form.
- Concentrate on your breathing and try not to hold your breath.

Fittest Variations:

If you can't support your weight, try an assisted parallel-bar dip. Most gyms have machines that have assistance levers you step on to help support your weight. For a real challenge, add a weight hooked around your waist. This will really give your triceps a pump.

Chair Dip

(Home Version of Parallel-Bar Dip)

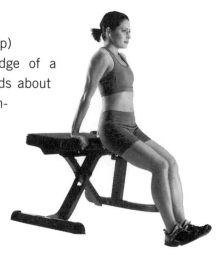

Starting Position. • Sit at the edge of a bench or chair. Position your hands about shoulder-width apart with your fingers facing forward, palms facing down, and elbows straight at your side. Place your legs straight in front of you with your body weight supported on your heels.

The Movement. • Lower your body toward the floor for two counts by bending your elbows, forming a 90-degree angle. Keep your back close to the bench. Pause, then return slowly for four counts to the starting position.

TRAINING TIPS:

- Your back should be as close to the bench as possible.
- Make sure that your elbows bend directly backward throughout the movement, otherwise you'll be putting an extra strain on your shoulders.
- Because you're using your own weight, this is a great activity to do anywhere, using a desk in your office, a bench in the park, or a ledge at the shopping mall.

Fittest Variations:

If you want to increase the difficulty of the activity, place your feet on another bench or chair rather than the floor. In this position your triceps will be working harder against the force of gravity. And if you want a real power blast, place a weight across your lap to increase the resistance even more.

BICEPS

Regular Dumbbell Curl
(Gym/Home Version)

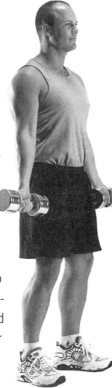

Starting Position. • Stand with your feet about shoulder-width apart, knees slightly bent, chest out, and head up. Grip a dumbbell in each hand. Your arms should be extended directly at your side and your palms facing forward.

The Movement. • Lift both dumbbells for two counts toward your shoulders. Your elbows should be closely fixed to your side. Pause, then slowly lower the dumbbells for four counts back to the starting position.

TRAINING TIPS:
- Your wrists should be in a fixed position throughout the movement to avoid the weight from swinging around.
- Keep your abdominals tight.

Fittest Variations:
Alternate one arm, then the other. You can also try sitting on a bench instead of standing.

Hammer Curl

(Gym/Home Version)

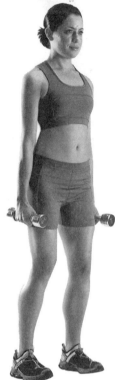

Starting Position. • Stand with your feet about shoulder-width apart, knees slightly bent, chest out, and head up. Grip a dumbbell in each hand, letting your arms hang directly at your side with your palms facing inward.

The Movement. • Lift both dumbbells directly up toward your shoulders for two counts. Your elbows should be close to your side. Pause, then slowly lower for four counts back to the starting position.

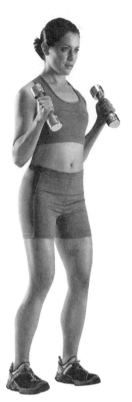

TRAINING TIPS:

- The movement should feel like you're using a hammer, but make sure to keep your elbows by your side through the entire movement.
- Keep your torso and abdominals tight to prevent your body from swinging back and forth.
- This is a great forearm developer.
- Standing against a wall can really help you maintain good posture throughout the movement.

Fittest Variations:

If you want, you can alternate one arm and then the other. You can also perform the activity sitting. If you do, make sure that your back stays straight without arching.

Concentration Curl

(Gym/Home Version)

Starting Position. • Sit on the edge of a bench or chair. Your legs and feet should be spread a little bit more than shoulder-width apart. Grip a dumbbell in your right hand, palm facing outward. Extend your arm and brace your elbow against the inside of your right thigh. Your left arm should be resting comfortably on your left leg.

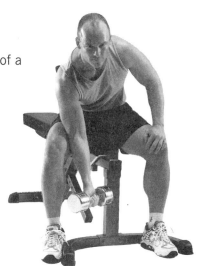

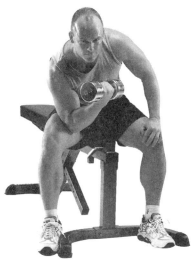

The Movement. • Keeping your elbow completely fixed against your leg, slowly curl the dumbbell for two counts up toward your shoulder while squeezing the bicep (feeling a little pump in the muscle). Pause, then slowly lower for four counts back to the starting position.

TRAINING TIPS:

- If you're just starting out, avoid taking the weight all the way down. The most important part is the "pump" when you curl your arm.
- Make sure the weight you're using isn't too heavy. If it is, it will cause you to arch your back and lower your shoulder, straining your lower back.
- Keep your arm fixed against your leg throughout the entire movement.

QUADRICEPS

Dumbbell Squat

(Gym/Home Version)

Starting Position. • Stand with your feet about shoulder-width apart, knees slightly bent, chest out, head up, and toes turned out just a bit. Grip a dumbbell in each hand. Your arms should be straight by your side with your palms facing inward.

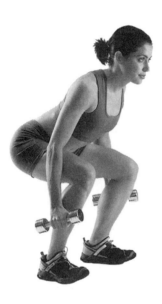

The Movement. • Slowly lower your body for four counts, pushing your hips and buttocks backward until your upper thighs are just about parallel with the floor. Keep your focus straight ahead, rather than turning your head up or down. Pause, then push through your upper leg and buttocks for two counts, returning to the starting position.

TRAINING TIPS:

- The trick to this activity is keeping your torso and abs tight so that you don't strain your lower back.
- For maximum benefit, don't lock your knees in the starting position.
- It helps to focus your eyes on one spot on the wall and keep your head up through the whole movement.
- Squats are a great butt-toner activity.
- To avoid knee damage, don't bounce.

Leg Press

(Gym Version)

Starting Position. • Sit on the cable leg press machine. With your back firmly against the padding, place your feet about shoulder-width apart. Adjust the machine so that your knees are at a 90-degree angle. Grip the handles with both hands.

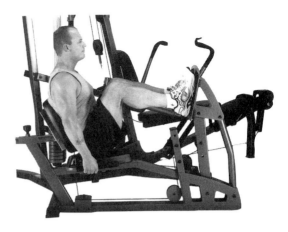

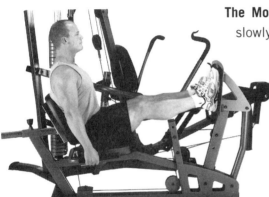

The Movement. • Push your legs slowly for two counts until they are almost completely straight. Keep your knees in line with your toes and drive through your heels. Pause, then slowly return for four counts to the starting position.

TRAINING TIPS:

- When straightening your legs, don't lock your knees.
- When you're lowering your legs back to the starting position, keep constant pressure on the cable and don't let the weights touch.
- Keep your head flat on the padding throughout the movement.
- This is a great butt firmer.
- If your gym doesn't have a cable leg press, you can also use a plate-loaded leg press.

Fittest Variations:

You can vary this activity by changing the position of your feet. You can widen your stance greater than shoulder width. You can also place your feet higher on the platform so that your toes are almost off the edge.

Stationary Lunge

(Home Version of Leg Press)

Starting Position. • Stand with your left foot about two to three feet in front of your right. Bend your left leg slightly, with your foot firmly on the ground. Your back leg should have a slight bend with your heel off the floor and your weight on your toes. Keep your hands comfortably by your sides, your head up, chest out, and back straight.

The Movement. • Lower your body for four counts until your right knee is al-most touching the floor and your left knee is bent as close to 90 degrees as possible. You should feel the muscle in your front thigh working hard. Pause, then keeping your torso straight up, press your front foot into the floor and slowly raise your body for two counts, back to the starting position. Complete your repetitions and then repeat with the right leg in front. When you finish both sides, that's one set.

TRAINING TIPS:

- Keep your chest lifted throughout the movement and don't let your back collapse. This will keep the pressure off your lower back.
- The position of the knee is important to watch out for. Don't let the knee drop below 90 degrees or move forward past your toes.
- To prevent knee injury, don't bounce at the bottom of the movement.

Fittest Variation:

When you can perform the movement with little or no difficulty, you can begin to add weights. Hold the dumbbells by your side or up on your shoulders.

Leg Extension

(Gym Version)

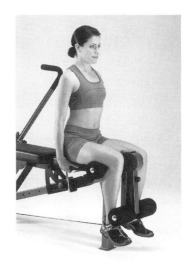

Starting Position. • Sit in the leg extension machine and adjust the back so that your knees fit comfortably over the front edge of the seat. Next, adjust the leg pads so that they comfortably rest on your shins, a little above your ankles. Grip the sides of the seat or the handles to prevent your hips from rocking back and forth.

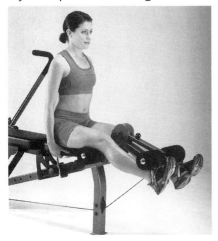

The Movement. • Raise both your legs for two counts until they are almost straight, with just a slight bend in your knees. Pause, then slowly lower for four counts, back to the starting position.

TRAINING TIPS:

- You shouldn't feel stress on your knees when you perform this activity. Be careful; flexing your knees beyond 90 degrees at the starting position can put a strain on them.
- Throughout the movement, keep your back completely against the padding and your thighs and butt fully on the seat. If your back moves away from the padding, you probably need to adjust the machine.

Fittest Variation:

You can do one leg at time if you want to focus on each muscle more fully. Remember, you'll be using less weight if you do each leg separately.

Dumbbell Leg Extension

(Home Version of Leg Extension)

Starting Position. • Sit on the end of a bench or chair with your back straight and head up. Make sure your legs are high enough off the ground so that they can bend 90 degrees. Place a dumbbell between your feet.

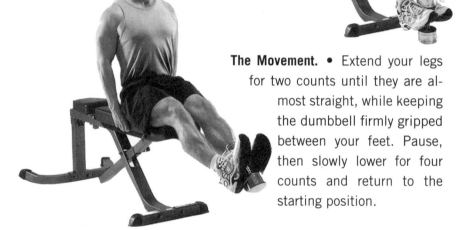

The Movement. • Extend your legs for two counts until they are almost straight, while keeping the dumbbell firmly gripped between your feet. Pause, then slowly lower for four counts and return to the starting position.

TRAINING TIPS:

- Hold on to the side of the chair or bench to help keep your hips from lifting.
- When you're lowering the dumbbell, resist the weight as much as possible, since you'll have gravity on your side. You should feel the muscle contract both on the way up and on the way down.

HAMSTRINGS

Straight-Leg Dumbbell Deadlift

(Gym/Home Version)

Starting Position. • Stand with your feet about shoulder-width apart, knees slightly bent, chest out, and head up. Grip two dumbbells with your palms facing inward. Your arms should be extended straight in front of you, touching your thighs.

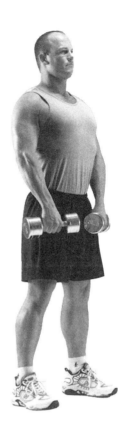

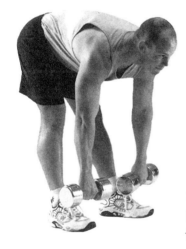

The Movement. • Bending at your hips, *slowly* lower the dumbbells for four counts toward your feet. Pause, then raise the dumbbells for two counts back to the starting position.

TRAINING TIPS:
- Pull your shoulders back at the starting position if they get rounded.
- If you feel pain in your lower back, stop the activity.
- To prevent serious back injury, don't bounce at the bottom of the movement.

Lying Leg Curl

(Gym Version)

Starting Position. • Lie facedown on the leg curl machine. Adjust the roller pads to a position right above your heels. Your knees 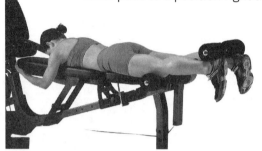 should be just off the bench. Grip the hand bars near your head to help keep your upper body and hips in contact with the padding.

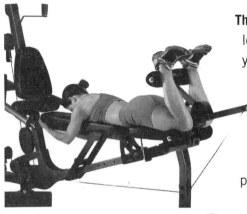 **The Movement.** • Curl your legs for two counts toward your buttocks. Try to bring your heels as close to your butt as possible. Pause, then slowly lower your legs for four counts, back to the starting position.

TRAINING TIPS:

- Keep your hips and thighs down throughout the entire movement to avoid putting too much stress on your lower back.
- Strong hamstrings help to keep your leg muscles balanced. We tend to focus on the front thigh muscles and ignore the weaker back hamstring muscles.

Fittest Variations:

Alternate one leg, then the other, so that you can focus more fully on the muscle. Point your toes up during the movement to intensify the work of your hamstrings.

Dumbbell Leg Curl

(Home Version of Lying Leg Curl)

Starting Position. • Lie facedown on a bench. Place a dumbbell between your feet and grab the sides of the bench to hold yourself in position.

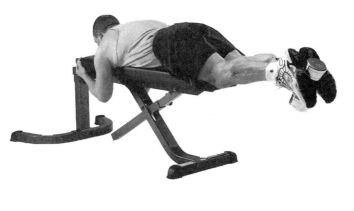

The Movement. • Curl your feet toward your butt for two counts so that the dumbbell is as close to touching as possible. Pause, then slowly lower your legs for four counts and return to the starting position.

TRAINING TIPS:

- It will take some practice to grip the dumbbell between your feet while lying on the bench. Try placing the dumbbell on the floor right next to your legs and carefully grab it with your feet. Even better, have your friend or spouse help you out the first couple of times. You may also want to start with a low weight until you get the hang of the movement and can keep the dumbbell from falling.
- When you're lowering the weight, you'll have gravity on your side, so focus on keeping your hamstring completely contracted.

Dumbbell Lunge

(Gym/Home Version)

Starting Position. • Stand with your feet about shoulder-width apart, knees slightly bent, chest out, and head up. Grip two dumbbells and hold them directly at your side with your palms facing inward.

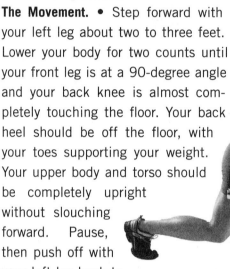

The Movement. • Step forward with your left leg about two to three feet. Lower your body for two counts until your front leg is at a 90-degree angle and your back knee is almost completely touching the floor. Your back heel should be off the floor, with your toes supporting your weight. Your upper body and torso should be completely upright without slouching forward. Pause, then push off with your left leg back to

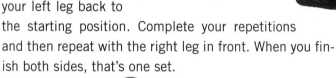

the starting position. Complete your repetitions and then repeat with the right leg in front. When you finish both sides, that's one set.

TRAINING TIPS:

• This is a difficult movement to do properly. I suggest practicing without any weight until you can maintain the form consistently through ten to twenty repetitions.

• To prevent straining your knee, don't let your knee extend over your toes.

Fittest Variation:

Instead of staying in one position you can perform the movement by walking across the room. This only works if you have a space that's big enough to do at least ten continuous lunges. If you do this variation, remember you'll be doing right and left at the same time.

One-Leg Dumbbell Calf Raise

(Gym/Home Version)

Starting Position. • Place the ball of your right foot on a step, block, or telephone book with your heel hanging off the edge. Grip a dumbbell in your right hand, letting it hang down at your side with your palm facing inward. Hook your left leg behind your right leg or just raise it off the ground slightly behind you. For support, place your left hand against a wall or other object to keep yourself steady.

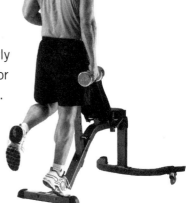

The Movement. • Press up on your right toe as far as possible, feeling a stretch in the back of your calf. Pause, then slowly lower your leg for four counts back to the starting position. Complete your repetitions, then repeat with the other leg. When you finish both sides, that's one set.

TRAINING TIPS
- Your back should be as straight as possible and your lifting leg slightly bent throughout the movement.
- As you lift your leg up, don't let your foot roll forward.
- Remember to switch the dumbbell to the same side as the lifting leg.

Fittest Variations:

To work the inside part of your calf, you can angle your leg 45 degrees outward. To work the outside part of your calf, angle your leg 45 degrees inward.

ABDOMINALS

Regular Crunch

(Gym/Home Version)

Starting Position. • Lie flat on your back with your knees bent and your feet flat on the floor. Your feet should be about a foot from your hips. Comfortably place your hands across your chest.

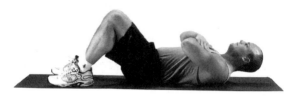

The Movement. • Flatten your lower back against the floor. At the same time, use your abdominal muscles to slowly raise, for two counts, your head and shoulders off the floor about a foot. That's as far as you need to go. Pause, then lower down for two counts to the starting position, without completely touching the floor.

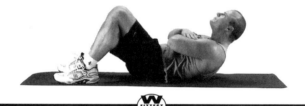

TRAINING TIPS:

- This is a difficult movement to do correctly so that you're just working your ab muscles. Most importantly, keep your back flat on the floor and chin off your chest.
- Feel your abs contract each time you complete the movement. After a few repetitions you should feel a burning sensation in your abs, which means you're doing the movement correctly.

Fittest Variations:

You can try placing your feet on a bench or chair. To make the movement even more challenging, you can place a small weight or dumbbell on your chest.

Elbow-to-Knee Crunch

(Gym/Home Version)

Starting Position. • Lie on your back with your knees bent about hip-width apart and your feet flat on the floor. Place both hands behind your head and your fingers lightly touching.

The Movement. • Lift your right shoulder off the floor for two counts, aiming to touch your right elbow to your left knee. Pause, then slowly lower for two counts and re-turn to the starting position. Complete your repetitions, then repeat on the left side. When you finish both sides, that's one set.

TRAINING TIPS:

- Keep your neck relaxed throughout the movement. Don't pull or twist your neck.
- For maximum benefit use a slow, controlled motion.

Fittest Variations:

Place your left ankle on your right knee and keep your right foot on the floor. Do the same movement trying to touch right elbow to left knee. You'll feel a little more of a stretch. Reverse this leg position for the other side.

In the starting position, keep your left leg straight. Bring your left knee toward your right elbow. Reverse this leg position on the other side.

Reverse Crunch

(Gym/Home Version)

Starting Position. • Lie on your back with your hands directly by your sides, palms facing down. Bend your knees at a 90-degree angle so that your thighs are perpendicular and your lower legs almost parallel to the floor. Your ankles should be touching.

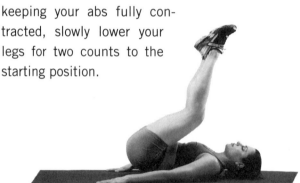

The Movement. • Lift your hips up off the floor, pulling your knees toward your chest for two counts. Your hips should raise only a few inches off the floor. Pause, then, keeping your abs fully contracted, slowly lower your legs for two counts to the starting position.

TRAINING TIPS:
- Don't swing your hips around, but keep them very controlled throughout the movement.
- Keep your neck flat on the floor and avoid the temptation to lean forward to look at your legs. This keeps you from straining your neck muscles.

Fittest Variation:

Hold a dumbbell between your feet to add resistance.

Side Crunch

(Gym/Home Version)

Starting Position. • Lie on your back on the floor or a mat, with your knees bent. Drop your knees by twisting them to the left. Your right knee should be directly above the left. Place your hands so they're lightly touching the back of your head and both shoulders are firmly touching the floor.

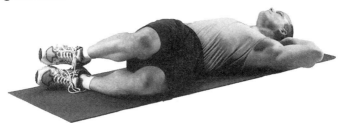

The Movement. • Raise your head and shoulders off the floor for two counts by contracting only your ab muscles. Pause, then slowly lower for two counts and return to the starting position. Complete your repetitions and then repeat on the other side. When you finish both sides, that's one set.

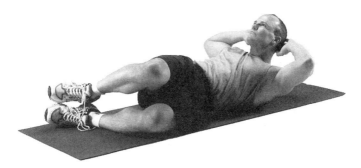

TRAINING TIPS:

- Believe it or not, the movement is very small and concentrated. You don't need to lift your shoulders as far as they can go, only enough so that you feel it in the side and abdominal muscles.
- Keep your neck from twisting and turning up toward your body.
- This is great for toning your love handles and obliques.

APPENDIX C:
STRETCHING

Seated Toe Touch

Starting Position. • Sit on the floor with your legs straight in front of you.

The Movement. • Bending slowly at your hips, reach forward to touch your toes. Hold and then release.

The Feeling. • You should feel the stretch in the back of your legs.

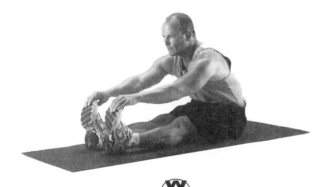

STRETCHING TIPS:
- Don't worry if you can't reach your toes; most people can't. Just reach as far as you can go.
- For an added stretch, place a towel around your feet and pull yourself forward.

Hurdle Stretch

Starting Position. • Sit on the floor with your right leg extended straight forward and your left leg bent so that the left foot is touching the right knee.

The Movement. • Keeping your right leg straight, bend from your hips. Reach both your arms toward your right foot, grabbing the toes of the foot or holding on to the bottom of your lower leg. Hold and then release. Repeat on the other side.

The Feeling. • You should feel the stretch in the back of your right leg and through your hip.

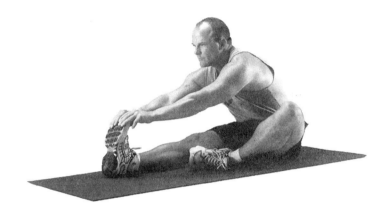

STRETCHING TIPS:

- If you can't reach your toes, you can wrap a towel around your extended leg to help you stretch.
- Make sure your extended leg has a slight bend, don't lock out your knee.

Straddle Stretch

Starting Position. • Sit with your legs straight and open as far apart as you can.

The Movement. • Reach your right hand to your left foot. Hold and then release. Reach your left hand to your right foot. Hold and then release. Reach both hands as far forward in front of you as you can. Hold and then release.

The Feeling. • You should feel the stretch in the back of both your legs and your lower back.

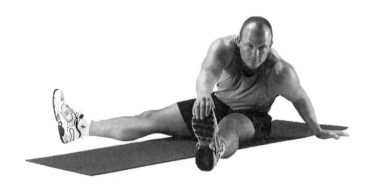

STRETCHING TIPS:
- Move slowly from your right to left side.
- Keep your neck relaxed throughout all the movements.

Seated Groin Stretch

Starting Position. • Sit on the floor with your body erect. Place the soles of your feet together about two feet in front of you and your knees dropping out to the side.

The Movement. • Place your hands on your ankles and slowly lean forward, using your elbows to gently push down your knees. Try to touch your nose to your feet. Hold and then release.

The Feeling. • You should feel the stretch on your inner thighs and pelvis.

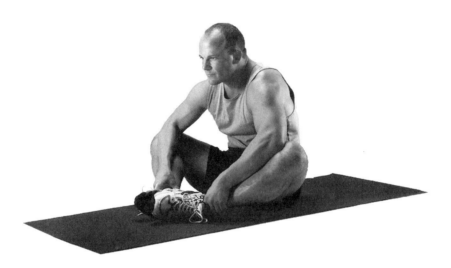

STRETCHING TIPS:
- Keep your back straight throughout the movement.
- Don't force your knees to the floor with your elbows.

Standing Quad Stretch

Starting Position. • Stand straight up with your legs together. Place your left hand on a chair or the wall for support.

The Movement. • Bend your right leg. Reach back with your right hand and grab hold of your right foot. Gently pull your foot toward your butt as far as you can without feeling a strain. Hold and then release.

The Feeling. • You should feel a stretch in the front of your upper leg.

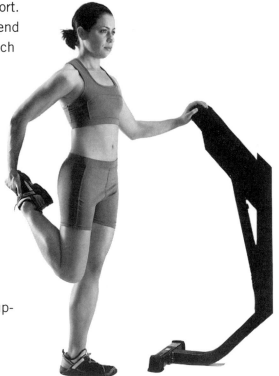

STRETCHING TIPS:
- Keep your knees together.
- Stand tall through entire movement and don't lean forward.

Calf Stretch

Starting Position. • Stand with your right leg in front of your left leg about two to three feet. Place both your hands against a wall or chair about shoulder height.

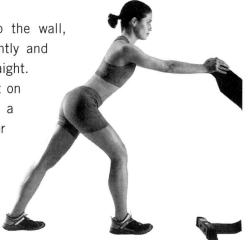

The Movement. • Lean into the wall, bending your right leg slightly and keeping your left leg straight. Your left heel should be flat on the floor. You should have a straight line from your lower left leg through your back. Hold and then release. Switch legs.

The Feeling. • You should feel the stretch in the back of your calf.

STRETCHING TIPS:

- Make sure to keep your hips and toes facing forward.
- If you don't feel enough of a stretch, move your back leg farther away from the wall.
- Keep the heel of your back leg flat on the floor.

Chest Stretch

Starting Position. • Stand with your legs about shoulder-width apart and your arms by your sides with palms facing inward.

The Movement. • Bring your arms behind your back, interlocking your fingers. Pull your arms straight away and up from your body. Hold and then release.

The Feeling. • You should feel the stretch across your chest and through your shoulders.

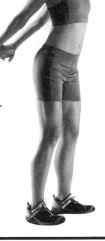

STRETCHING TIPS:

- Keep your shoulders down when you raise your arms behind your back.
- If you're having trouble interlocking your hands, hold on to a towel instead.
- Look straight ahead, keeping your neck relaxed.

Overhead Triceps Stretch

Starting Position. • Stand with your feet about shoulder-width apart. Raise your right arm and place it behind your head in the small of your back with your elbow bent.

The Movement. • Place your left hand on your right elbow. Gently push down on your right elbow. Hold and then release. Repeat with your other arm.

The Feeling. • You should feel a stretch in the back of your right arm.

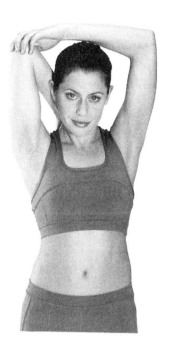

STRETCHING TIPS:
- Make sure to maintain good posture throughout the stretch.
- Keep your neck relaxed.

Wrist Extensor Stretch

Starting Position. • Stand with your legs about shoulder width apart. Raise your right arm up straight in front of you with your palm facing upward.

The Movement. • With your left hand, grasp your right fingertips from the palm side and gently pull them back toward your body. Hold and then release. Repeat with your other arm.

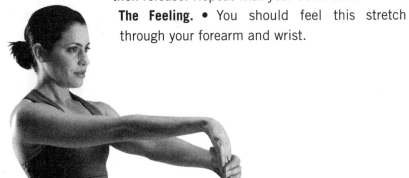

The Feeling. • You should feel this stretch through your forearm and wrist.

STRETCHING TIPS:

- This is a great stretch to do at the office to help prevent carpal tunnel syndrome. Try using it after typing at the computer every few hours.
- Don't pull too far back; that will overstretch the muscle.

Back Extension/Cobra

Starting Position. • Lie on your stomach on the floor in a sort of push-up position. Your hands should be by your sides underneath your shoulders with your palms facing down and fingers pointed forward.

The Movement. • Push through with your hands to lift just your upper body off the floor (head, shoulders, and chest only). Keep your pelvis on the floor and your head looking forward. Hold and then release.

The Feeling. • You should feel your spine lengthen and release.

STRETCHING TIPS:

- Don't just press back with your hands, push your upper body up and forward.
- Keep your head looking forward. Tilting your head back to look at the ceiling will strain your neck.

Cross Shoulder Stretch

Starting Position. • Stand tall with your legs about shoulder-width apart. Extend your right arm across your chest so that it's parallel to the floor at shoulder level. Place your left hand on the back of your right elbow.

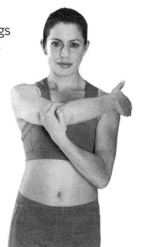

The Movement. • Gently press your right arm into your body and across your chest. Hold, then release. Repeat with the other arm.

The Feeling. • You should feel the stretch through your right shoulder.

STRETCHING TIPS:
- Keep your shoulders relaxed; don't shrug them.
- This is a great stretch for helping to prevent shoulder injury.

Chin-to-Chest Stretch

Starting Position. • Stand with your legs about hip-width apart and your arms hanging loosely by your side. Look straight ahead.

The Movement. • Gently tilt your neck forward, tucking your chin to your chest. Hold and then look all the way up.

The Feeling. • You should feel a stretch in the back of your neck, lengthening and releasing tension.

STRETCHING TIPS:
- Keep both shoulders pressed down.
- This is a great stretch to release tension if you're stressed out.

Ear-to-Shoulder Stretch

Starting Position. • Stand with your legs about shoulder-width apart and your arms hanging loosely by your side. Look straight ahead.

The Movement. • Gently tilt your neck to the left so that your left ear is toward your shoulder. Hold and return to the starting position. Repeat on the other side.

The Feeling. • You should feel a stretch in the left side of your neck.

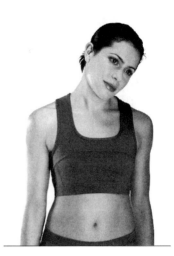

STRETCHING TIPS:

- Maintain good posture and only tilt your neck, not the rest of your body.
- This is an excellent stress reliever.

APPENDIX D:
RECIPES

These recipes are some of my favorites. Nothing too fancy, just the basics. Most of them you can prepare in less than twenty minutes. For some of them you'll have to add more time for cooking. If you're working out at home, you might want to put the meat loaf in the oven first, then do your workout. That's one trick I use if I'm short on time. You'll also see that most of the recipes have many servings. This will also save you time. Freeze your leftover servings in small, individual plastic containers. When you want it again for dinner, just pop it in the microwave to defrost it. In no time you'll have a hot, delicious meal.

Yes, these are recipes that have helped me become the World's Fittest Man—which I cook myself at home. But, I've refined them for you to try at home with the help of nutritionist Heather Greenbaum. With her expertise you can be sure you're getting the perfect combination of nutrients to fuel your body and flavor to whet your appetite. Be sure to let me know which ones you like best by e-mailing me on my Web site.

World's Fittest Man Power Pasta Primavera

MAKES 4 SERVINGS

3 cups cooked whole-wheat pasta, any type

4 chicken breast halves (about 4 oz. each), skinned, boned, and all visible fat removed

⅛ tsp. salt

⅛ tsp. pepper

1 tbsp. olive oil

1 garlic clove, finely chopped

1 large carrot, cut into julienne strips

1 cup broccoli florets

1 cup cauliflower florets

1 can (10.75 oz.) low-fat cream of chicken soup

½ cup skim milk

¼ cup nonfat Parmesan cheese

Directions

1. Cook the pasta al dente according to package directions.

2. While pasta is cooking, rinse chicken with cool water, and pat it dry with paper towels. Cut the chicken into one-inch strips. Sprinkle the chicken with salt and pepper; set aside.

3. Heat olive oil in a nonstick skillet over medium-high heat. Add garlic and chicken strips. Cook and stir for about 4 minutes or until the chicken is no longer pink inside. Remove the chicken and place in a bowl to keep warm. Do not drain oil from skillet.

4. In same skillet, sauté carrots, broccoli, and cauliflower for 5 minutes over medium heat. Add cream of chicken soup, skim milk, Parmesan cheese. Cook, uncovered, over low heat until vegetables are tender, about 10 minutes.

5. Stir in chicken and pasta.

One Serving:
Calories: 385; Fat: 8.4 g; Protein: 35 g; Carbohydrates: 41 g

World's Fittest Man Super Stir-fry with Chicken

MAKES 4 SERVINGS

1 lb. chicken breast halves, skinned, boned, and all visible fat removed; cut into one-inch pieces

4 tbsp. reduced-sodium soy sauce

1 tsp. ground ginger

1 tsp. olive oil

1 garlic clove, finely chopped

1 cup broccoli florets

1 cup cauliflower florets

1 carrot, chopped

4 green onions, chopped (green part only)

¼ cup low-sodium chicken broth

¾ cup mandarin oranges, drained

Directions

1. Mix 2 tbsp. soy sauce and ginger in a small bowl. Add chicken and marinate for 10 minutes. If you want you can marinate for longer. Simply cover bowl with plastic wrap and refrigerate for desired time (the longer you marinate the better the flavor).

2. Heat olive oil in a nonstick skillet over medium heat. Stir in garlic, then add chicken and marinade together. Cook and stir for about 4 minutes or until the chicken is no longer pink inside.

3. Add broccoli, cauliflower, carrot, and green onions. Cook and stir for about 2–3 minutes. Add chicken broth and remaining soy sauce; cover and steam 3–5 minutes.

4. Remove from heat and stir in oranges; serve.

One Serving:

Calories: 174; Fat: 2.6 g; Protein: 21 g; Carbohydrates: 19 g

World's Fittest Man Fabulous Chicken Fajitas

For the marinade:
2 tbsp. reduced-sodium soy sauce
½ tsp. ground ginger
1 garlic clove, finely chopped
2 tbsp. olive oil
1 tbsp. ground cinnamon
⅓ cup chopped fresh cilantro
1 pinch chili powder
½ tsp. hot pepper sauce
4 tbsp. fresh lime juice

To finish the dish:
4 chicken breast halves (about 4 oz. each), skinned, boned, and all visible fat removed, sliced diagonally into strips
1 jalapeño, chopped
1 cup sliced red onions
1 green pepper, cut into julienne strips
1 red pepper, cut into julienne strips
4 large whole-wheat flour tortillas, 9-in. diameter
1 cup store-bought tomato salsa
½ cup low-fat sour cream

Directions

1. Combine all marinade ingredients in a shallow baking dish and mix well. Add chicken and toss until well coated. Marinate for 15 minutes.

2. Coat nonstick skillet with nonstick spray. Cook and stir the jalapeño, red onions, and green pepper over moderate heat for 5 minutes. Stir in chicken and cook, uncovered, until chicken is tender and no longer pink.

3. Warm the tortillas by wrapping in foil and heat in the oven at 325 degrees.

4. Serve chicken on warm tortilla and top with salsa and sour cream.

One Serving:
Calories: 364; Fat: 9.7 g; Protein: 33 g; Carbohydrates: 45 g

World's Fittest Man Awesome Turkey Meatloaf

MAKES 8 SERVINGS

1½ lb. ground turkey
  (90 percent lean)
½ cup tomato juice
2 tbsp. tomato paste
½ cup rolled oats

2 egg whites
½ cup chopped onions
½ tsp. oregano
½ tsp. salt
¼ tsp. pepper

Directions

1. Preheat oven to 350 degrees.
2. Mix ground turkey, tomato juice, tomato paste, rolled oats, egg whites, onion, oregano, salt, and pepper in a large bowl. Mix thoroughly.
3. Coat a 9" x 5" x 3" pan with nonstick spray and press the mixture into pan.
4. Bake for 50–60 minutes or until meat thermometer at center reads 175 degrees.

One Serving (1 slice):
Calories:158; Fat: 7.4 g; Protein: 17 g; Carbohydrates: 5 g

World's Fittest Man Salmon Teriyaki

MAKES 4 SERVINGS

½ cup reduced-sodium soy sauce

2 tbsp. cooking sherry, dry or sweet

1 tbsp. grated fresh ginger

2 garlic cloves, finely chopped

1 tbsp. brown sugar or honey

4 salmon steaks (4 oz. each)

Directions

1. Combine all ingredients except salmon in small bowl. Wisk until completely blended.
2. Place salmon in baking pan and coat with marinade. Cover with plastic wrap and refrigerate up to one hour. Turn the salmon occasionally to completely absorb the marinade.
3. Preheat oven to 350 degrees. Bake salmon in marinade for 10 minutes or until flakes easily when tested with a fork.

One Serving:
Calories: 204; Fat: 6.8 g; Protein: 25 g; Carbohydrates: 8 g

World's Fittest Man Lemon Grilled Salmon with Spicy Sweet Potato Sticks

For sweet potato sticks:

1 tbsp. olive oil

½ tsp. paprika

½ tsp. salt

1 tsp. hot pepper sauce

4 medium-size sweet potatoes, sliced lengthwise into quarters

Directions

1. Preheat oven to 400 degrees. Use nonstick spray for baking sheet.
2. Whisk together olive oil, paprika, salt, and hot sauce in a large mixing bowl. Add sweet potatoes and mix by hand until completely coated.
3. Place sweet potatoes in single layer on a large baking sheet coated with nonstick spray.
4. Bake for 40 minutes.

For the salmon:

4 salmon steaks (4 oz. each)

¼ tsp. salt

juice of 1 lemon (about 3 tbsp.)

Directions

1. Coat unheated grill with nonstick spray.
2. Cover salmon with salt and lemon juice and place on grill.
3. Cook salmon for about 4 minutes on each side, until browned and flakes easily when tested with a fork.

Fittest Variations:

If you don't have a grill you can broil the salmon in your oven broiler. And if you're short on time, poke a few holes in the sweet potatoes with a fork and cook for 5–8 minutes in your microwave.

One Serving (Salmon and Sweet Potatoes):

Calories: 270; Fat: 7.6 g; Protein: 24 g; Carbohydrates: 25 g

World's Fittest Man Sweet Shepherd's Pie

MAKES 6 SERVINGS

1 lb. sweet potatoes, peeled and quartered

1½ lb. ground turkey (90 percent lean)

1 large onion, finely chopped

1 garlic glove, finely chopped

¼ cup store-bought low-fat spaghetti sauce

1 bay leaf

1 tsp. chili powder

1 tsp. thyme

½ tsp. tarragon

¾ cup low-sodium vegetable broth

1 tbsp. of dry red wine or cooking sherry

1 cup chopped cauliflower

2 large carrots, chopped

1 cup chopped broccoli

⅓ cup skim milk

1 tsp. salt

Directions

1. Preheat oven to 350 degrees.
2. Boil sweet potatoes in a large saucepan over high heat for 20 minutes or until tender with a fork. Drain and return to saucepan.
3. While potatoes are cooking, coat a nonstick skillet with nonstick spray. Brown ground turkey with onion and garlic over medium heat.
4. Stir in spaghetti sauce, bay leaf, chili powder, thyme, and tarragon. Mix in vegetable broth and red wine. Add cauliflower, carrots, and broccoli. Simmer uncovered until most of the liquid is cooked off and vegetables are tender, not mushy. Remove bay leaf.
5. To cooked potatoes, add skim milk and salt; mash with a fork or potato masher until smooth. Add pepper to taste.
6. Spoon meat mixture into an ungreased 10" x 10" x 2" baking dish. Spread mashed potatoes over the surface; use a fork for texture. Bake for 30 minutes, or until lightly browned on top.

One Serving:
Calories: 293; Fat: 9.9 g; Protein: 23 g; Carbohydrate: 27 g

World's Fittest Man
Dijon Mustard Chicken Nuggets

MAKES 4 SERVINGS

2 tbsp. Dijon mustard
1 tbsp. low-fat mayonnaise
½ cup skim milk

1 lb. chicken breast halves, skinned, boned, and all visible fat removed; cut into one-inch pieces
1 cup crushed bran flakes
¼ tsp. salt

Directions

1. Preheat oven to 425 degrees.
2. Coat a baking pan with nonstick spray.
3. Whisk Dijon mustard, low-fat mayonnaise, and skim milk until smooth, without lumps in a small bowl. Stir in chicken.
4. Mix bran flakes and salt in a separate bowl. Dip each piece of chicken from milk mixture into flakes until completely coated. Place coated chicken on the baking pan.
5. Bake 8–12 minutes, until chicken is tender and no longer pink.

One Serving:
Calories: 221; Fat: 9.8 g; Protein: 20.2 g; Carbohydrates: 14 g

World's Fittest Man Paella with Brown Rice

MAKES 4 SERVINGS

1 clove garlic, finely chopped
½ lb. chicken breast halves, skinned, boned, and all visible fat removed; cut into one-inch pieces
1 can (14.5 oz.) low-sodium chicken broth
½ can (28 oz.) peeled and diced tomatoes

¼ tsp. saffron
1 cup brown rice, uncooked
½ lb. fresh or frozen shrimp, shelled and deveined (thaw shrimp if frozen)
salt and pepper to taste

Directions

1. Coat the bottom of a unheated large saucepan with nonstick spray. Over medium heat, add garlic and stir. Add chicken; cook and stir for 2–3 minutes, until lightly browned on the outside.
1. Pour in chicken broth, tomatoes, and saffron. Bring to a boil, then reduce and simmer covered over low heat for 10 minutes.
2. Add brown rice; stir completely. Simmer, covered, about 30 more minutes, or until rice is almost tender.
3. Add shrimp and simmer, covered, for 5 more minutes until shrimp, chicken, and rice are tender.

One Serving:
Calories 262, Fat: 2.3 g; Protein: 21 g; Carbohydrates: 38 g
Fittest Variation:
You can make this recipe using all chicken or shrimp.

World's Fittest Man Black Bean and Turkey Chili

MAKES 8 SERVINGS

1½ lb. ground turkey (90 percent lean)

1 onion, diced

2 cans (15.5 oz.) black beans, drained

2 cans (14.5 oz.) reduced-sodium Italian-style stewed tomatoes

1 package (1.25 oz.) reduced-sodium chili or taco seasoning mix

1 can (4 oz.) green chili peppers, chopped

1 can (8 oz.) tomato sauce

Directions

1. Coat the bottom of a large saucepan with nonstick spray.
2. Cook and stir ground turkey and onion over medium-high heat until meat is brown and no longer pink. Drain any excess liquid.
3. Stir in black beans, stewed tomatoes, chili seasoning mix, green chili peppers, and tomato sauce. Heat to a boil; reduce to low-medium heat and simmer covered for 20–30 minutes.

One Serving (1 cup):
Calories: 285; Fat 7.6 g; Protein: 23 g; Carbohydrates: 31 g

World's Fittest Man White Bean Salmon Cakes

MAKES 6 SERVINGS

For the salmon cakes:
1 can (14.75 oz.) pink salmon,
    drained
½ can (15.5 oz.) white beans, drained
¾ cup crushed bran flakes
½ chopped fresh parsley
2 tbsp. lemon juice
2 egg whites
1 tsp. hot pepper sauce

¼ tsp. paprika
¼ tsp. salt
1 tbsp. vegetable oil

For the sauce:
1 cup diced cucumber
1 cup plain low-fat yogurt
2 garlic cloves, finely chopped
½ tsp. dried dill weed

Directions

1. Remove visible bones and skin from salmon. Blend salmon and white beans with a potato masher in a mixing bowl until white beans are completely mashed. Mix in bran flakes, parsley, lemon juice, egg whites, hot pepper sauce, paprika, and salt.
2. Shape mixture into 6 patties.
3. Heat vegetable oil in a nonstick skillet on medium-high heat. Cook patties for 4 minutes on each side until golden brown.
4. Combine sauce ingredients in small bowl. Mix thoroughly.
5. Serve salmon cakes topped with cucumber yogurt sauce.

One Serving (1 patty and sauce):
Calories: 210; Fat: 7.7 g; Protein: 21 g; Carbohydrates: 15 g

World's Fittest Man Catfish Creole

1 cup brown rice, uncooked
1 can (14.5 oz.) reduced-sodium
   Italian-style stewed tomatoes
1 small onion, chopped
1 tsp. chicken bouillon granules

½ tsp. oregano
¼ tsp. garlic powder
¼ tsp. hot pepper sauce
1 lb. catfish fillets, cut into one-inch
   pieces

Directions

1. Cook brown rice according to package directions.
2. Combine stewed tomatoes, onion, chicken bouillon granules, oregano, garlic powder, and hot pepper sauce in a medium saucepan over medium heat. Bring to a boil. Stir in catfish fillets.
3. Cook for 5–8 minutes or until catfish flakes easily when tested with a fork.
4. Serve over brown rice.

One Serving:

Calories: 365; Fat: 10.2 g; Protein: 23 g; Carbohydrates: 45 g

Fittest Variation:

You can use another type of flaky white fish such as bass or fillet of sole, if you prefer.

ACKNOWLEDGMENTS

I would like to thank my mom and dad for their never-ending support; my brother Greg for helping me through many races; Sam and Pete for being my brothers; my Grandmother Smysor for pushing me to dream; Uncle Ron for being a friend; all my family that has supported and followed me; Rick Kuplinski and Mike Yoder for helping me through those grueling races; Christina for supporting and putting up with me that year; all you Body Construction clients; Brad, CB, Pete, Brian, and Steve for always being there to drink beers and smoke cigars afterward; Karen for her continued support; my angels Susan, Marcy, and Judy for being my number-one fan club; Cathy, Loren, and the other incredible professors at WIU; Coach Mowery for helping get me started; my teachers at Cuba High and grade school; the New Orleans crew; all my Cuba and Fulton County friends; Sue and Alena for the calls; Brad A. for always being a friend; the gang at Attitudes; Ben for my first adventure race; Steve S. for keeping me out of trouble; my literary agent Joelle Delbourgo for making this happen; Eric for doing most of the work; my editor Amy Hughes for making this seem so easy; Daphne Howard and Denise Austin for getting my career started; Heather Greenbaum for her awesome nutrition expertise; Jennifer Elice for researching and writing about all those challenges;

James Pacello for editing and proofreading many drafts; Dana Mirmam for her press releases; Ken Kidd for endless ideas; Mitchel Gray for his beautiful workout photographs; Kristen Gambell, our very fit model; Peter Gregory for helping format; Sylvia Neuhaus for last-minute proofreading; and special thanks to Art Carey, Barry Gringold, Peter Neuhaus, Robert Kempe, Amanda Kain, Tracey Budz, Geralyn Lucas, Al Roker, Linell Smith, Brian Tart, Anna Cowles, Kathleen Schmidt, and Meredith White.

Finally, Greg Jenkins, Bill Wagner, Leon Southwick, and my many other friends who have passed away but have made their mark on my life; and the thousands of wonderful people who I have come in contact with over the years and who have enriched my life so much. If I have missed anyone, I apologize. Thank you all so much!

INDEX

ABOUT THE AUTHORS

Joe Decker is recognized as "the World's Fittest Man," an ultra-endurance power athlete, renowned fitness trainer, and syndicated columnist who has helped thousands of women, men, kids, and seniors get into shape and lose weight.

Joe believes in leading by example and is a personal testament to overcoming addictions and obstacles. Once overweight and out of shape, Joe transformed his body and his life through an amazing journey from fat to fittest. In 2000 he broke the *Guinness World Records* 24-Hour Physical Fitness Challenge to help inspire and motivate people to get fit.

Joe has appeared on *The Today Show, Discovery Health, The Early Show, The O'Reilly Factor,* and Fox News and has been featured in *The Washington Post, The Philadelphia Inquirer, The Baltimore Sun, Men's Fitness, Muscle and Fitness, Men's Health,* and *GQ.* To his surprise, *People* magazine named him one of America's 50 Most Eligible Bachelors in 2000.

In addition to breaking the world fitness record, Joe has competed in many of the world's toughest endurance and adventure fitness events. Some of these include the Raid Gauloises, the Badwater 135, the Marathon des Sables ("The World's Toughest Footrace"), the

Grandslam of UltraRunning, the Tough Guy Challenge in England, and the Empire State Building Run-Up race in New York City.

After serving three years in the army with the 10th Mountain Division, Joe graduated from Western Illinois University with a bachelor of science degree in exercise science. He founded his own innovative fitness company working with individuals, groups, and corporate clients. Joe is regularly involved in charity work. He has established a scholarship program and research foundation for childhood obesity at Western Illinois University from his winnings on *The Weakest Link*. He lives and works in the Washington, D.C., area. Visit him at his website Joe-Decker.com.

Eric Neuhaus is a writer, journalist, and former television producer for *ABC News* and *20/20*. He lives and works in New York City.

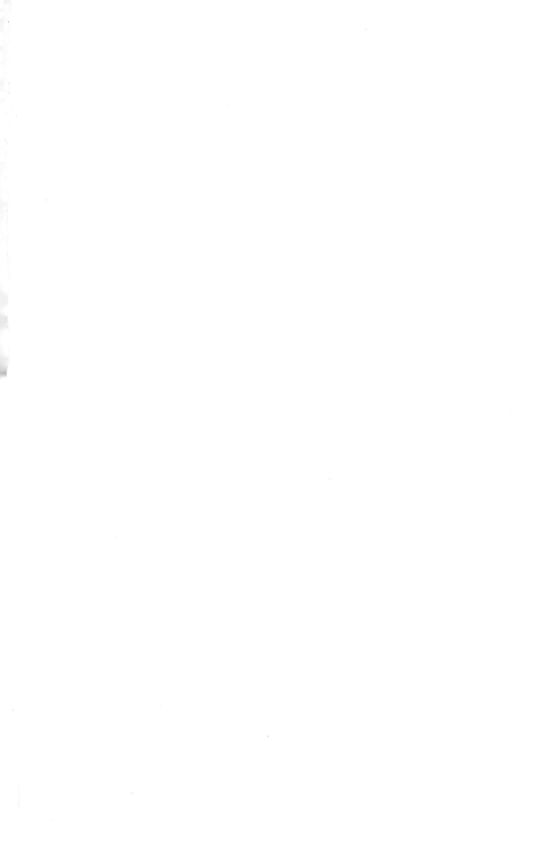